PRESCRIPTION DRUG ENCYCLOPEDIA
New, Expanded Edition

By Gayle Cawood, M.Ed., Janice McCall Failes,
and Frank W. Cawood

Acknowledgements

This book is the result of many loving, caring people who want to make it easier for you to know how prescription drugs can affect you and your body.

To our friend Cheryl Daly, for your patience, accuracy, and dedication: we thank you.

To our physician and pharmacist friends: thank you for your concientious reading of our text and your invaluable suggestions.

To the loving staff of FC &A, for being understanding and available: we thank each one of you.

To our families, who loved us and encouraged us: we thank you.

But most of all, our thanks and praise is for our Lord and Saviour, Jesus Christ, who loves and directs us.

It was you who created my inmost self,
And put me together in my mother's womb;
For all these mysteries I thank you;
For the wonder of myself,
For the wonder of your works.
You know me through and through,
From having watched my bones take shape
When I was being formed in secret,
Knitted together in the limbo of the womb.
                                        -Psalm 139: 13-15

Your body, you know, is the temple of the Holy Spirit, who
is in you since you received Him from God. You are not
your own property; You have been bought and paid for.
That is why you should use your body for the glory of God.
                                        -1 Corinthians 6: 19-20

(Quotations from **The Jerusalem Bible**)

TABLE OF CONTENTS

PREFACE

PUBLISHER'S NOTE

The authors have diligently attempted to provide up-to-date and accurate information in this book. However, with the rapid advances that medical and biochemical research make daily, it is recommended that you, the consumer, contact your pharmacist or physician regarding the most current information on any specific drug. Don't hesitate to ask questions of those who prescribe your medicine or fill your prescriptions. It is your body and life they seek to heal, and each person's body can react differently to drugs, because drugs are chemicals.

Since pharmacology — the science of drugs — is such a rapidly expanding field, the publisher cannot be responsible for the results of any drug therapy program undertaken by anyone who has consulted this book for information. This publication does not constitute medical practice or advice. Its only intent is to provide the consumer with easy-to-understand information.

Please consult carefully with your physician before taking any drugs or before discontinuing any medication.

1

WHAT'S IN THIS BOOK?

Most people have taken medicines to fight infection, to ease pain, to aid in getting to sleep, or to be helped to feel better. Many individuals don't ask questions about the prescriptions their doctors give them. They take medicine and await its good effects — the effects that the doctor intends it to have. Unfortunately, prescription drugs often have troublesome side effects.

This book will provide you with up-to-date, easy-to-understand information about the most frequently prescribed drugs: their intended effects and their possible side effects. **This book should be an encouragement to you to communicate openly with your physician and pharmacist.** In order to be treated successfully, a patient needs to know what to tell the doctor, especially facts about previous or present drug reactions or problems. Any new or unusual ache, discomfort or physical or mental sensation should be reported at once to your doctor. He cannot fully do his job if he does not have complete information from you.

The terms "generic" and "brand name drug" are explained in *Chapter 2.* Doctors and pharmacists across the country are questioning the quality of generic drugs that the FDA has approved. You, the consumer, need to know exactly what "generic" means.

Chapter 3 discusses common matters of safety which

9

are of concern whenever medicines are taken. The importance of following the prescribed dosage to avoid overdoses, possible hazards to the unborn or nursing child from drugs, and suggestions to protect yourself against tampered drugs are all mentioned. Also, information about storing drugs properly and a few rules for taking medicine are provided.

Many people don't know exactly what questions they need to ask their doctors or druggist. *Chapter 4* gives some basic guidelines for asking and answering questions, so that you and your doctor will have the information which is necessary for proper medication prescribing.

Chapter 5 highlights the information on drugs that is presented in this particular book, in detail in *Chapter 6*. Each drug entry will contain information on the "Category of Drug", its "Intended Effects", its reported "Side Effects", with additional "Warnings" or "Possible Interactions" described.

The main part of the book, of course, is *Chapter 6*. Each drug, whether a brand name or a generic name, is listed in alphabetical order. Where appropriate, several brand name and generic drugs have been cross-referenced and included under a complete drug class entry. Several brandname medicines consisting of two specific drugs have been cross-referenced to those two main drugs.

Over 700 of the most frequently prescribed drugs are presented. All of these drugs have been tested thoroughly by their manufacturers and have been approved by the FDA. Their described effects and side effects have been documented by thousands of studies.

At the end of the book, two additional sections are provided as extra sources of information. A simple **Glossary** of many medical terms and symbols is provided. And, there is a list of complete names and addresses of the major **Drug Manufacturers**, in case you want to contact them for further information.

We trust that the particular format of this book will make

10

it easy for you to find out the facts about your medicines. Also, we hope that our efforts at "translating" medical vocabulary into everyday language will make the facts understandable to you.

WHAT ARE "GENERIC DRUGS"?

All drugs are chemicals, either occurring naturally or manufactured. All medicines which your doctor prescribes can be described by either of three possible names:

1. A chemical name
2. A generic (general) name
3. A trademarked brand name

The **chemical** name precisely lists the exact chemical ingredients in that drug. Usually, only manufacturers and pharmacists use this description. The **generic** name is a type of abbreviation for the common name of a drug's main ingredient. Most often, a medicine can be prescribed by its **brand name.** This is the specific, trademarked name given to a particular ingredient or special combination of ingredients which one manufacturer is marketing.

Generic names of drugs are not trademarked, so two different manufacturers can use the same drug, make it into different sized and colored pills, and call the same ingredient by two different brand names. Strict government standards are supposed to mean that differences in quality between competing generic drugs will be small. However, some generics, particularly antiseizure and antipsychotic drugs, aren't as effective as their brand name equivalents because of differences in particle size or the use of different fillers that may interfere with absorption. Your doctor's using a generic name when writing a prescription could save you money, because one manufacturer's version of "**Medicine X**" often costs more than another manufacturer's version.

For example, if your doctor decides you need treatment with penicillin (a broad, generic name for a class of drugs), he could prescribe either of these generic names for you, depending on the type of penicillin he believes is best:

amoxcillin

or

penicillin V.

Or, he could be more specific and use, for example, one of these brand names for that particular type of penicillin:

Generic / Brand Names:

Amoxcillin / Amoxil ® or Larotid®

Penicillin V / Pen-Vee-K® or V-Cillin K®

Some drugs which have been developed by a single manufacturer contain a particular ingredient or special combination of ingredients. If no other manufacturer produces this same ingredient or combination of ingredients, that brand name drug may not have a generic equivalent available; in other words, it is only available by its brand name.

If you take a certain medicine regularly, check with your pharmacist to see if that drug is available generically. If it is, ask if there would be any savings in having your doctor prescribe it under its generic name.

Also, ask the pharmacist if he will substitute the lowest priced generic drug for the drug named on your prescription (if it isn't the lowest priced.) Most states have laws allowing pharmacists to do this without your doctor's approval.

In *Chapter 6*, brand name drugs which are available generically have been cross-referenced to the generic drug. Likewise, in the information on generic drugs, many of the specific brand names which are most frequently prescribed are listed.

14

3

WHY ARE PRESCRIPTION DRUGS DANGEROUS?

As the drug manufacturers recommend, you should contact your doctor immediately if you experience any of the possible side effects mentioned in this book. If the side effects are greater than expected, he will then decide whether to change your dosage, to change to another drug, or perhaps to discontinue the medication. Just as you should never *take* a prescription drug without a doctor's consent, you should never *stop taking* medication a doctor has prescribed without consulting him. Serious problems can continue without proper medication, just as other problems can arise from discontinuing medication.

OVERDOSES ARE DANGEROUS

Whenever your physician prescribes a medicine for you, he has an intended purpose in mind and has designated a specific dosage of that drug for you. *Deadly* results can occur from taking more than the doctor prescribes. Do not try to "hurry up" the good effects of the medicine by increasing the recommended dose. Chemicals take a while to work within the body to bring about desired results. Give them time.

If accidental overdosage should occur, contact your doctor

immediately. If hospital or ambulance emergency care is required, give the medical personnel the medicine bottle, so they can respond properly. If the bottle is not available, tell them the exact name and dosage of the drug and the name of the doctor who prescribed it.

PREGNANCY AND DRUGS

During pregnancy and while breast-feeding, whatever affects the mother's body and biochemical system will probably affect the baby. A woman requiring medicines during pregnancy should advise the doctor of her condition. The physician must then weigh the possible hazards to the baby against the benefits to the mother, and he must decide what is best for them both.

Most doctors recommend that *pregnant or nursing women should not take any unnecessary drugs, to avoid any possible danger to the child.* Some drugs have been found by their manufacturers to cause moderate to severe birth defects.

Drugs may be required to maintain the mother's health. The main objective of any medical treatment is to have as healthy a mother as possible and as healthy a baby as possible. Information on a particular medicine's side effects and your doctor's advice will determine the best means to ensure the health of both mother and child.

PROTECT YOURSELF AGAINST TAMPERED DRUGS

Since the recent threats of tampering against several name brand, non-prescription drugs, all consumers must learn to protect themselves against being victims of drug tampering.

Although over-the-counter drugs have been carefully

packaged and are strictly regulated by the federal government, there is no foolproof way to keep the drugs entirely safe. To protect you and your family, follow these guidelines, recommended by the U.S. Pharmacopoeial Convention.

1. Before you buy:

~Consider what form the product that you are buying is available in — and buy the form that is least likely to be sabotaged. A tablet or caplet is more difficult to tamper with than capsules or liquids.

2. While you're buying:

~Carefully inspect the outer packaging of the product. Do not purchase it if it looks at all unusual.

~Compare the box or container you choose with others of the same product. Make sure there is nothing different about the package you buy.

3. When opening the package:

~Watch for holes, tears, cracks or breaks in the outer wrapping, cover or protective seal.

~Check to see if the outer covering has been changed, unwrapped, or replaced.

~Read the lot number and information on the box or outer covering, and make sure that it matches the information on the product label or container.

~Inspect the shrinkband seal around the top of the container to see if it has been stretched, distorted or opened and retaped.

~If it is an unsealed bottle, make sure the cap is on very tightly.

~Check that the bottle is filled properly and not overfilled or underfilled.

~Is there a seal in place?

~Look at the cotton plug or filler at the top of the container. Make sure it hasn't been disturbed.

~Inspect the inside rim of the container for bits of paper or glue — this may mean that it formerly had a protective seal under the cap.

4. While taking the medicine:

~Make sure the color, smell, consistency and moistness of the product are what you are used to.

~Take the medicine in good lighting so you can double check that it has not been tampered with, and that it is the proper drug for your ailment.

Do not take any drug that doesn't seem just right. If you are suspicious about a drug or find any evidence of tampering, contact your local office of the FDA (Federal Drug Administration) or your pharmacist — right away.

STORING PRESCRIPTION AND NON-PRESCRIPTION DRUGS CORRECTLY

With several different prescriptions to take each day, people have been looking for ways to make it easier to store their drugs. But drugs are chemicals that can be harmed or changed by the way they are stored. Here are some important things to remember about how you store your medicine.

1.) Drugs should always be kept in the container the pharmacist supplies. Some pills must be protected from light, and some will be damaged by contact with air or moisture. If the bottle or container the pharmacist gives you is too large, just ask for another container that is more convenient for you. Don't store drugs in a regular pill box. Some drug manufacturers are introducing their own pill containers — patients can use these and be secure that their pills will not be harmed.

2.) Do not put different kinds of pills in the same container. Putting different types of pills together can create chemical reactions and changes. They can form harmful substances or become inactive. It is tempting to put your pills in little plastic boxes that have separate compartments for each day and different times — but if your pills become inactive they will not do you any good. Also, when drugs are combined in the same container, people often forget which pill is which.

3.) Watch for changes in color, smell or consistency in your drugs. If you notice any such changes, take them to your pharmacist. He will be abe to tell you whether they are still safe to take. For example, when aspirin develops a vinegary odor, it has probably lost its potency and should not be used.

4.) Watch the expiration date. This date is good only when the bottle *has not been opened*. Many drugs decompose when they are exposed to air. Once the seal is broken on a bottle, the expiration date is *no longer* in effect. Ask your pharmacist or doctor how long the drug is good after the bottle is opened. Then, when you open it, write your own expiration date on the bottle. For example, nitroglycerin is potent for only 3 months after it has been exposed to air.

5.) If possible, avoid storing medicines in the bathroom. Since moisture and heat are the worst enemies of most drugs, the medicine cabinet in the family bathroom is *not* the best place to store them. The dampness from showers and baths can harm the potency of your drugs. Try to choose a safe, dry and cool place to store your prescription and non-prescription drugs.

6.) Use easy-to-open bottles. Many over-the-counter drugs come in child-proof containers that are sometimes "adult-proof". Especially if you have arthritis, those bottles can be hard to open. If you are sure that children will not be near your drugs, ask your pharmacist for a container that is easy to open.

7.) Keep all medicines out of the reach of children. If you have children at home or will have little ones visiting your house, be sure to keep all drugs where the children will not be able to get to them.

SIX RULES FOR TAKING MEDICINE

Over one billion prescriptions are written by physicians every year. An article in the Journal of the American Medical Association (JAMA), revealed that 78% of these prescriptions were being taken improperly. Sometimes it is the doctors who do not take enough time to explain their instructions, but many patients disregard the instructions that they do receive. The following guidelines will help ensure that you get the best results from your medicine.

1.) Inform your doctor or pharmacist of any medication you are already taking: this also includes any daily vitamin or mineral supplements, as well as any non-prescription drugs (aspirin, cold medicines, etc.) that you take regularly. Many drugs interact with each other and lose or gain potency or cause serious side effects when taken together.

2.) Keep track of any side effects you may experience while taking prescription drugs, and report them to your doctor.

3.) Do not drink alcohol while taking any medicine, unless you have your doctor's approval. Alcohol may cause serious interactions with some drugs or increase side effects of many others.

4.) Always follow the label instructions; if there is a difference between your doctor's verbal instructions and the label instructions, contact your doctor immediately. There are good reasons why some medicine is to be taken with food, or needs to be refrigerated or shaken well before using. If you don't follow these instructions, your medicine may be useless or even harmful to you.

5.) Unless your doctor tells you otherwise, take ALL of the prescribed medicine. Just because you feel better doesn't mean you are completely well. Also, some medicine is prescribed to prevent certain problems. But, whether your medicine is for prevention or cure, always take it as directed.

6.) Never take drugs prescribed for someone else. Drugs

are prescribed on the basis of other drugs being taken, one's age, weight, health history, and other factors. Exchanging medicine is dangerous.

4

WHAT DO I NEED TO ASK MY DOCTOR OR PHARMACIST?

Your doctor and your druggist are your best resource people for any concerns or questions you may have about your medicines. Be sure your physician knows about all other medications you are taking, both prescribed drugs and non-prescriptive medicines (such as: aspirin, laxatives, cold medicines, etc.). Also tell him about any drug-related reactions or problems you may have had. Your pharmacist can answer questions about medical terms and drug interactions. Futhermore, the drug manufacturers themselves have people on staff eager to provide you with information or hear from you about drug-caused reactions.

If you don't ask, you may not find out. And what you don't know could prevent you from alerting people who can help you.

QUESTIONS TO ASK ABOUT YOUR PRESCRIPTION DRUGS

The National Council on Patient Information and Education says up to half of all drugs are taken improperly. The main reason for mistakes, according to the Council, is that people ask too few questions about the drugs their doctors prescribe.

Here are some guidelines of what to ask your doctor when

medication is prescribed for you or someone in your family:
. What is the name of the drug?
. What is it supposed to do?
. How long will it take before it is effective?
. How am I supposed to take it?
. When am I supposed to take it?
. When should I stop taking it?
. Are there any foods, drinks, other drugs or activities that I should avoid while taking this drug?
. What are the drug's side effects?
. What should I do if the side effects happen to me?
. Is written information available on this drug that I could have?
. How can I get this written information?

A PRESCRIPTION LIST COULD SAVE YOUR LIFE

Keep a list of all your current prescriptions in your wallet, billfold or purse. Include the name of the drug, what dose you are taking and the doctor's name who prescribed it. When you visit your doctor (or doctors) have them check your list and keep it up to date. The list will remind your doctor (or doctors) of all your current prescriptions and could help avoid dangerous drug interations. During an emergency, the list will provide valuable information at the doctor's fingertips.

Taking time to learn more about prescriptions can help ensure that:

1.) you are taking your drugs properly so they will be most effective

2.) you will know if something unusual occurs

3.) you will know what your doctor wants you to do if something unusual happens.

5

HOW IS INFORMATION ABOUT DRUGS PRESENTED IN THIS BOOK?

CHAPTER 6 contains the core of this book. More than 700 different drugs are listed alphabetically. Many are trade-marked, brand name drugs. Others are listed under their generic or general names. Several are grouped under their general drug class.

In order to provide complete yet concise drug descriptions, the authors have chosen not to fill up pages unnecessarily with repetitious information. For example, both Lopressor® and Inderal® are "beta-blockers". Their intended effects, side-effects and possible problems are quite similar. So, instead of including the same lengthy information under each of these brand names, they have been grouped together and described in detail under one drug class entry — Beta-Adrenergic Blocking Agent Class. Thus, when looking up information about Inderal®, you will find a reference to **See: Beta-Adrenergic Blocking Agent Class.**

CROSS-REFERENCES

There are two types of entries found in *Chapter 6:* cross-references and main entries. Brand names or generic drugs which are described fully elsewhere, under a common main entry, will have a "**See**" reference. This will direct you to the main entry for that drug, where the complete information is provided. Also, each cross-reference of a brand name drug will list its "**See**" reference information with manufacturer's name in parentheses, so you can write them for their latest product information, if you need to.

MAIN ENTRIES
The name of the manufacturer of each brand name drug is given in parentheses. For example, Darvon® is manufactured by the Eli Lilly drug company; it will be listed as:

Darvon® (*Lilly*)

Brand names are designated with a registered trademark sign ®, such as *Darvon®*. Generic (or general) names of drugs will not have a specific manufacturer noted, since several different drug companies may produce medicines with that generic name.

Generic/Brand Names:
This section lists all drugs found in this book which are in the same class. It is not a complete listing of all generic or brand name drugs which are available, just the most frequently prescribed drugs, which appear in this book. Thus, under a particular class of drugs, for example "Penicillins", the *Generic / Brand Names* will be listed as follows:

Amoxcillin / Amoxil ® or Larotid®
Penicillin V / Pen-Vee-K® or V-Cillin K®

Category of Drug:
This describes the general purpose of a particular drug. One medicine may be for high blood pressure (Blood Pressure Reducer), while another may be to fight infection (Antibiotic). These terms, and many others, are found fully explained in the last chapter, the *Glossary*.

Ingredients:
This information gives the generic names for the ingredients found in particular brand name drugs. You may know if you have an allergy or sensitivity to a certain chemical or drug. By knowing what a newly prescribed drug contains, you can avoid possible serious reactions.

Intended Effects:
This will answer your questions as to why your doctor has given you a certain medication. The "good" results of the drug will be described in this section.

Side Effects:
The side effects described may be quite unlikely, with less than a 1% chance of occurrence in many cases. Do not assume that you will suffer from any of the side effects, just because many undesirable side effects are listed.

Manufacturers are required by law to advise the consumer of any and all types of adverse reactions which people have reported in response to taking their medications. Some of the side effects are natural, expected and unavoidable. Most of the side effects listed are unusual, unexpected and quite infrequent. The side effects may also be dosage-dependent; many times they will lessen or completely disappear if the dosage is lowered or as your body adjusts to taking the medicine -- but consult your doctor before changing your intake of the medicine.

The listing of the side effects is an effort to help you be a better-informed patient. If you know what the possible side effects of a drug may be, you will be better able to report your condition and your reactions to your doctor.

As the manufacturers suggest, *if any of the known side*

effects do occur, notify your doctor immediately. He can then best decide how to continue your treatment. *Do not stop taking any prescribed medication without your doctor's opinion.* Sometimes he will switch you to another medicine. But, sometimes it may be best for you to put up with some minor discomfort caused by the drug, because the medicine's intended effects outweigh its side effects. Keep your doctor informed. If he fails to be responsive to your problems, seek another physician's advice.

Warnings:
This section alerts you to serious facts which have been noted about the drug. Notify your doctor immediately if any of the warnings apply to you.

Possible Interactions:
This information should help you realize the complex nature of the body, and how one drug can affect the action of another drug. Also certain dietary-intake problems have been noted, such as salt restriction, cautious use of alcohol, and certain foods which may change the effectiveness of drugs.

Note: No Rx prescription required
This note means that the U.S. Food and Drug Administration doesn't require a doctor's prescription for sale of a drug. Some states may make exceptions to this and require prescriptions for some drugs that the U.S. government thinks are safe to be sold without prescription.

PACKAGE INSERT
Remember, whenever you have a prescription filled, you can ask your pharmacist for the "package-insert" for that medication. This leaflet describes in medical language and

detail all known effects and side effects of that drug. If your druggist does not have the leaflet in stock, you can ask for the name of the drug's manufacturer and write to them for it. Manufacturer's addresses are provided at the end of *Chapter 6*.

6

ALPHABETICAL LISTING OF PRESCRIPTION DRUGS

Accutane® (*Roche Laboratories*)
See: Isotretinoin

ACE Inhibitors
See: Angiotensin Converting Enzyme Inhibitor Class

Acebutolol
See: Beta-Adrenergic Blocking Agent Class

Acetaminophen

Brand Names: Anacin-3®, Datril®, Panadol®, Phena-phen®, Tylenol®.

Category Of Drug: Pain Reliever, Fever Reducer

Intended Effects: To relieve mild to moderate pain, to reduce fever.

Side Effects: Drowsiness, skin rash. Rare: swelling of

31

vocal cords, hemolytic anemia, abnormally low white blood count, abnormal bruising or bleeding.

Warnings: Should be used with caution by patients with bronchial asthma or allergy to aspirin until sensitivity has been determined. Prolonged use in high doses by the elderly can cause liver damage with jaundice, anemia and kidney damage.

Possible Interactions: Slight possibility that acetaminophen may alter response to anticlotting drugs and increase the risk of abnormal bleeding.

Note: No Rx prescription required

Acetaminophen + Codeine

Brand Names:
Phenaphen® + Codeine, Tylenol® + Codeine

See: Acetaminophen
See: Codeine

Acetazolamide

Brand Name: Diamox®

Category Of Drug: Antiglaucoma, Diuretic

Intended Effects: To aid in treatment of certain kinds of glaucoma, to help control certain types of epilepsy, to reduce excessive fluid retention in the body.

Side Effects: Drowsiness, confusion, tingling feeling in the limbs, some loss of appetite, temporary nearsightedness.

Warnings: Not for people who have had an allergic reaction to any dosage of this drug, those with impaired kidney or liver function, or people with depressed sodium and/or potassium blood serum levels. Causes birth defects in animals--avoid during first three months of pregnancy. Safety for infants has not been determined. Do not exceed recommended dosage. Notify physician if skin rash, fever, nausea, diarrhea, headache, or ringing in the ears develop since this may indicate allergy to this drug. Patients who are allergic to sulfa drugs may also be allergic to this medicine.

Possible Interactions: Amphetamines and tricyclic antidepressants may cause increased effects. Acetazolamide may decrease the effects of lithium and aspirin.

Acetohexamide
See: Antidiabetic Class

Acetohydroxamic Acid

Brand Name: Lithostat ™

Category Of Drug: Urinary Tract Anti-infective

Intended Effects: To treat certain chronic urinary infections, to reduce levels of ammonia and alkaline in the urine.

Side Effects: Nausea, vomiting, loss of appetite, tiredness, anemia, headache, nervousness, tremors, upset stomach, skin rash, sensation of warmth, inflammation of the veins, depression, anxiety.

Warnings: Causes birth defects in animals — avoid during pregnancy. Women of child-bearing age should be counselled about using acceptable methods of contraception while taking Lithostat™. Should not be used by people with poor kidney function or inflammation of the veins.

Possible Interactions: Skin rash develops when taken with alcohol. Acetohydroxamic acid bonds to iron in the bloodstream; if supplementary iron is needed, injection into the muscles is the most effective method for the body to absorb it adequately.

Achromycin®V (*Lederle*)
See: Tetracycline Class

Actifed® (*Burroughs Wellcome*)

Category Of Drug: Antihistamine, Decongestant

Ingredients: Triprolidine + Pseudoephedrine

Intended Effects: To provide relief of symptoms of colds and nasal allergies, to help decongest nasal, throat, sinus and respiratory membranes, to neutralize the body's production of histamine. May be a more effective treatment for some patients who do not respond to drugs containing only antihistamines, since it also contains a decongestant.

Side Effects: Sleepiness, dizziness, impaired coordination, upset stomach, thicker bronchial mucus, skin rash, dry throat and mouth, lowered blood pressure, headache, tiredness, restlessness, irritability, nausea, vomiting, diarrhea, constipation, tightness of chest, exaggerated sunburn.

Warnings: Should be used with considerable caution in patients who have: bronchial asthma, glaucoma-like high inner-eye pressure, overactive thyroid, cardiovascular disease, high blood pressure, stomach ulcers, urinary tract problems or menstrual irregularities. Known to be present in mothers' milk — avoid drug or avoid nursing. When taken by children, mild stimulation is often noted.

Possible Interactions: May interfere with the action of high blood pressure medicines and MAO inhibitor antidepressants. Sedation may increase when taken with: tranquilizers, antihistamines, antidepressants, sedatives, sleep inducers, alcohol and narcotics.

Note: No Rx prescription required

Actifed-C®Expectorant (*Burroughs Wellcome*)

Category Of Drug: Anticough, Phlegm Loosener, Decongestant, Antihistamine

Ingredients: Codeine + Triprolidine + Pseudoephedrine + Guaifenesin

Intended Effects: To provide relief from both "wet" and "dry" coughs caused by colds or allergies, to act as a phelgm loosener in aiding the "coughing-up" of mucus in the chest, to aid in drying up the excess mucus in nasal and sinus passages, to neutralize the body's production of histamine.

Side Effects: Sleepiness, dizziness, impaired coordination, stomach upset, thicker bronchial mucus, skin rash, dry throat and mouth, lowered blood pressure, headache, tiredness, restlessness, irritability, nausea, vomiting, diarrhea, constipation, tightness of chest.

Warnings: As with any drug containing codeine, drug dependence can result with overuse. Should be used with considerable caution in pressure, over-active thyroid, heart or blood vessel disease, high blood pressure, stomach ulcers, urinary tract problems or menstrual irregularities. Known to be present in mothers' milk — avoid drug or avoid nursing. When taken by children, mild stimulation is often noted.

Possible Interactions: May interfere with the action of blood pressure reducers and MAO inhibitor antidepressants. Sedation may increase when taken with: tranquilizers, antihistamines, antidepressants, sedatives, sleep inducers, alcohol and narcotics. Non-prescription cough, cold or allergy medicines may interact unfavorably.

Note: See Codeine

Acyclovir -Topical (in a polyethylene glycol base)

Brand Name: Zovirax®

Category Of Drug: Antivirus

Intended Effects: To treat herpes simplex and initial genital herpes.

Side Effects: Discomfort, mild pain, stinging and burning of the skin, itching, rash, inflammation of the vulva.

Warnings: Not for use by those allergic or sensitive to acyclovir. Only use on the skin. Avoid contact with the eyes. May cause birth defects — avoid during pregnancy. Ointment should thoroughly cover all sores. Use a rubber glove or finger cover to apply ointment to prevent spread of infection. Do not exceed the recommended dose.

Possible Interactions: None known.

Adapin® *(Pennwalt)*
  See: Tricyclic Antidepressant Class

Adrenocorticoid Class - Systemic

Generic / Brand Names:
  Betamethasone
  Dexamethasone/Decadron®
  Flunisolide/Nasalide®
  Hydrocortisone
  Methylprednisolone/Medrol®
  Prednisone/Deltasone®
  Triamcinolone/Aristocort®, Kenalog®

Category Of Drug: Adrenal Hormone, Anti-inflammatory

Intended Effects: To supplement natural hormones (normally produced by the body's adrenal gland), to ease rheumatic disease (arthritis, bursitis,) to heal certain skin disorders, to control allergic reactions, to combat certain breathing problems or blood disorders, or to treat particular digestive or nervous system diseases. Provides relief of symptoms; does not necessarily cure the disease causing the

37

symptoms.

Side Effects: Fluid retention, muscle weakness, ulcers increased perspiration, easily bruised or slow-to-heal skin, dizziness, headache, menstrual irregularities, blood-sugar problems, glaucoma, inhibited growth in children, mood swings, sleeplessness, decreased resistance to infection.

Warnings: May mask signs of infection. Prolonged use may cause serious eye and nerve problems. Causes birth defects in animals — avoid during first three months of pregnancy. Known to be present in mothers' milk — avoid drug or avoid nursing. May cause lowered adrenal hormone production in children. Existing emotional or psychotic problems may be aggravated. Manufacturer recommends that the lowest dosage suitable for the disorder being treated be used, and that reduction in dosage be gradual. Dietary salt restriction and potassium supplements may be necessary. Do not stop taking medication suddenly. May reactivate tuberculosis. Causes upset stomach; doctor will prescribe antacids.

Possible Interactions: No food, beverage or alcohol interactions are expected. Heavy smoking may increase drug effectiveness, so caution is advised. Taking barbiturates may decrease effectiveness of this drug while increasing effects of the barbiturates. Adrenal hormones may decrease the effects of insulin or other antidiabetic drugs. Anticonvulsants may cause decreased effectiveness. Do not take with aspirin — may cause severe ulcers.

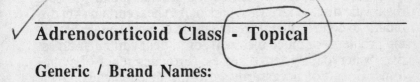

Adrenocorticoid Class - Topical

Generic / Brand Names:

Amcinonide/Cyclocort®
Betamethasone/Diprosone®, Valisone®
Desonide/Tridesilon®
Desoximetasone/Topicort®
Dexamethasone/Decadron®
Fluocinolone/Synalar®
Fluocinonide/Lidex®
Fluorometholone/FML® Liquifilm®
Flurandrenolide/Cordran®
Halcinonide/Halog®
Hydrocortisone/Hytone®, Westcort®
Methylprednisolone/Medrol®
Triamcinolone/Aristocort®, Aristocort A®, Kenalog®

Category Of Drug: Adrenal Hormone

Intended Effects: To provide relief and healing of in-flammed or irritated skin or eye conditions. Provides relief of symptoms; does not necessarily cure the disease causing the symptoms.

Side Effects: Burning, itching, irritation, dryness, acne-like breakout, skin discoloration, slight infection, weakening of tissue.

Warnings: If irritation worsens, contact your physician for other treatment. If large areas are treated, or if treatment continues for a long period of time, see **Warnings** and **Side Effects** listed under **Adrenocorticoid Class - Systemic,** because the body will be absorbing large amounts of the hormones applied to the skin. Certain brands of these creams are intended for use only in the eyes or only on the skin; do not use for any other purpose.

Albuterol

Brand Names: Proventil®, Ventolin®

Category Of Drug: Bronchial-Tube Relaxer

Intended Effects: To provide temporary relief of breathing difficulties in bronchial asthma, bronchitis and emphysema.

Side Effects: With large doses: bronchial fluid build up and inflammation, pounding heartbeat, dizziness, nervousness, nausea, heartburn, bad or unusual taste, dry mouth, vomiting, headache, insomnia, anxiety tension, excitation or blood pressure changes. Rare: dizziness, weakness, flushing of the skin, sweating, anginal-type chest or arm pain, ringing in the ears.

Warnings: Should be used with caution by people with high blood pressure, diabetes, overactive thyroid, coronary heart disease, congestive heart failure. If dizziness or chest pains occur, or if usual dosage does not improve condition, physician should be notified.

Possible Interactions: If taken with beta-blockers, effects of both drugs are diminished. If taken with epinephrine or other bronchial-tube relaxers, increased effects may result. Should be used with caution by people taking inhibitors or antidepressants to avoid changes in blood pressure. Should be used 20-30 minutes before taking beclomethasone dipropionate, to reduce potential toxicity.

Aldactazide® (*Searle*)

Category Of Drug: Diuretic, Blood-Pressure Reducer

Ingredients: Spironolactone + Hydrochlorothiazide

Intended Effects: To lower blood pressure, to promote elimination of sodium (salt) and water from the body; contains an ingredient which helps to minimize potassium loss, which often occurs when taking a diuretic. Often prescribed for patients with congestive heart failure, cirrhosis of the liver, essential hypertension, or fluid retention.

Side Effects: Fluid or electrolyte imbalances (signaled by: dry mouth and throat, weakness, drowsiness, restlessness, muscle cramps, low blood pressure, stomach distress), breast enlargement, blood-sugar problems, diarrhea, confusion, menstrual irregularities, excess hair growth, jaundice, dizziness, headaches.

Warnings: Potassium intake should be regulated upon physician's advice. Caution should be used when planning any type of anesthesia. Use with extreme caution in pregnant women — can interfere with development of the fetus. Known to be present in mothers' milk — avoid drug or avoid nursing. Salt intake should be under physician's guidance. As with other drugs containing thiazides, may activate or worsen lupus.

Possible Interactions: Do not take with triamterene. Large doses of aspirin may decrease its effects. Other blood-pressure reducers may increase the effects of this drug, as can barbiturates, MAO inhibitor antidepressants and pain relievers. If taken with digitalis careful monitoring and adjustments are required.

Note: See Thiazide Diuretic Class

Aldactone® (*Searle*)
See: Spironolactone

Aldoclor®(*Merck Sharp & Dohme*)
See: Methyldopa
See: Thiazide Diuretic Class

Aldomet® (*Merck Sharp & Dohme*)
See: Methyldopa

Aldoril® (*Merck Sharp & Dohme*)
See: Methyldopa
See: Thiazide Diuretic Class

Allopurinol

Brand Names: Lopurin®, Zyloprim®

Category Of Drug: Uric Acid Reducer

Intended Effects: To reduce the formation of uric acid, to combat gout, uric acid kidney stones and the deposit of uric acid products in the joints, bones and tissues by inhibiting an enzyme in the body which converts a type of protein (purines) into uric acid. To lower levels of uric acid in the blood which are raised by certain cancer treatments.

Side Effects: Most frequent: skin rashes. Less frequent;

hives, bleeding under the skin, peeling of skin and other skin disorders, loss of hair, nausea, vomiting, diarrhea, abdominal pain, damage to the liver and kidney, blood disorders, cataracts, fever, chills, low white blood cell count, itching.

Warnings: Notify physician immediately at first sign of skin rash since this may indicate allergy to the drug. Causes birth defects in animals — avoid during first three months of pregnancy. Known to be present in mothers' milk — avoid drug or avoid nursing. Do not take if close relatives have iron-storage disease.

Possible Interactions: Interacts with sulfinpyrazone, aspirin, acetaminophen and other drugs which affect uric acid metabolism. Thiazide diuretics and ethacrynic acid may interfere with the action of allopurinol. Allopurinol may prolong the activity of anticlotting drugs. Iron may accumulate in the body when taken in the form of iron supplements with allopurinol.

Alupent® (*Boehringer Ingelheim*)
  See: Metaproterenol

Note: Available in <u>Aerosal</u> or <u>Oral</u> forms

Amantadine

Brand Name: Symmetrel®

Category Of Drug: Antivirus, Antitremor

Intended Effects: To prevent and treat respiratory tract infections caused by influenza type A viruses, and to treat Parkinson's disease.

Side Effects: Most frequent: fear, faintness, depression, congestive heart failure, psychosis, urinary retention, hallucinations, confusion, irritability, loss of appetite, constipation, nausea, lightheadedness, fluid retention. Less frequent: dry mouth, headache, vomiting, fatigue, insomnia, sense of weakness. Infrequent: slurred speech, skin rash, visual disturbances. Rare: eczema, lowered white blood count and convulsions.

Warnings: Causes birth defects in animals — avoid during first three months of pregnancy. Known to be present in mothers' milk — avoid drug or avoid nursing. Parkinson's disease patients should not discontinue this drug abruptly. Should be used with caution by patients with liver disease, history of recurrent eczema rash, psychosis, congestive heart failure, fluid retention, low blood pressure, seizure disorders, kidney disease. Drive with caution if blurred vision occurs.

Possible Interactions: May increase the effects of levodopa, alcohol, sedatives and other antitremor drugs. Stimulants may increase the effects of amantadine.

Ambenyl® Expectorant (*Marion*)
　See: Antihistamine Class
　See: Codeine

Amcill® (*Parke-Davis*)

See: Penicillin Class

Amcinonide
See: Adrenocorticoid Class — Topical

Amiloride

Brand Name: Moduretic®

Category Of Drug: Blood-Pressure Reducer, Diuretic

Intended Effects: To lower blood pressure by eliminating excess fluid from the body. Specifically useful for patients who cannot take thiazide diuretics.

Side Effects: Nausea, loss of appetite, abdominal pain, gas, belching, mild skin rash, headache, weakness, tiredness, irregular heartbeats, diarrhea, stomach pain, elevated blood potassium levels, itching, leg aches, dizziness, difficult breathing, chest pain, back pain, increased heartbeat, constipation, upset stomach, changes in appetite, bloated feeling, hiccups, thirst, vomiting, gout, dehydration, flushing, muscle cramps, joint pain, numbness, stupor, loss of balance, inability to sleep, nervousness, depression, sleepiness, mental confusion, bad taste, visual disturbances, stuffy nose, impotence, difficult, painful, or involuntary urination, abnormal liver function, dry mouth, fever.

Warnings: Should not be used by people with poor kidney function, diabetes, high blood potassium levels, sensitive to sulfonamides, taking spironolactone or triamterene. Discontinue Moduretic® at least three days before glucose tolerance testing.

Possible Interactions: Thiazide diuretics will increase its effects. Do not use with lithium. Insulin requirements for diabetics may need to be adjusted. Known to be present in mothers' milk — avoid drug or avoid nursing. Take with food to avoid stomach upset. Drive or operate machinery with caution. Avoid large quantities of salt or salty foods.

Aminophylline
See: Xanthine Class

Amitriptyline
See: Tricyclic Antidepressant Class

Amoxapine

Brand Name: Asendin®

Category Of Drug: Antidepressant

Intended Effects: To relieve reactive or neurotic depressive disorders, psychotic depression, or depression accompanied by agitation or anxiety.

Side Effects: Blurred vision, clumsiness, shakiness or trembling, skin rash, itching, mental confusion in elderly patients, drowsiness, dry mouth, constipation, headache, nausea, nightmares. Rare: irregular heartbeat, fainting, vision changes, numbness, difficulty in urination, severe sunburn.

Warnings: Use with caution in people with history of seizures, glaucoma, urinary retention, heart problems. Discontinue treatment before surgery. Not recommended during the immediate recovery period for heart attack.

Possible Interactions: Not for people who are allergic to dibenzoxazepine compounds. Should not be given with MAO inhibitors since convulsions could result. May increase hazards of electroshock treatment if given at same time. Sedation may increase when taken with: tranquilizers, antihistamines, antidepressants, sedatives, sleep inducers, alcohol and narcotics.

Amoxicillin
See: Penicillin Class

Amoxil® (*Beecham*)
See: Penicillin Class

Amphetamine Class

Generic/Brand Name:
Dextroamphetamine/Dexedrine®

Category Of Drug: Stimulant

Intended Effects: To treat sleep epilepsy, to treat hyperactivity or restlessness in children. No longer recommended as an appetite suppressant.

Side Effects: Pounding or rapid heartbeat, high blood

pressure, over-stimulation, restlessness, dizziness, insomnia, euphoria, tremor, headache, dryness of the mouth, reduced growth in children, unpleasant taste, diarrhea, constipation, loss of appetite, weight loss, itching, changes in sex drive. Behavior changes or psychosis, especially with overdose.

Warnings: Amphetamines have a high potential for addiction — do not exceed recommended dose for any reason! Tolerance develops after a few weeks. Avoid increasing doses. Do not discontinue this drug abruptly to avoid withdrawal symptoms, extreme fatigue and mental depression. Drive and operate machinery with caution. Avoid in cases of advanced hardening of the arteries, heart disease, high blood pressure, overactive thyroid, glaucoma, sensitivity to other stimulants, previous history of drug addiction, mental illness and children under three. Causes birth defects in animals — avoid or use with extreme caution during pregnancy or while nursing.

Possible Interactions: May decrease the effects of guanethidine. If taken with or within 14 days of taking MAO inhibitor antidepressants, may cause high blood pressure. Tricyclic antidepressants may increase the effects of amphetamines. May alter insulin requirements of diabetics. Phenothiazines may decrease the effects of amphetamines.

Ampicillin
See: Penicillin Class

Anaprox® *(Syntex)*
See: Naproxen

Angiotensin Converting Enzyme (ACE) Inhibitor Class

Generic / Brand Names:
Captopril/Capoten®
Enalapril Maleate/Vasotec®

Category Of Drug: Blood-Pressure Reducer

Intended Effects: To reduce blood pressure and (Captopril only) to help manage heart failure.

Side Effects: Headache, dizziness, tiredness, diarrhea, low blood pressure, cough, nausea, faintness upon rising, chest pain, awareness of heartbeat, inability to sleep, tingling sensations, abdominal pain, vomiting, difficult breathing, swelling of the hands or feet, itching, rash.

Captopril only: Protein in the urine, kidney failure, urinary frequency, increased urine elimination, decreased urine elimination, deficiency of certain blood cells, reduction of blood platelets, joint pain, increased susceptibility to infections, fever, tongue ulcers, scalded mouth sensation, sensitivity to the sun, separation of the nails from the skin, loss of hair, increased heart rate, congestive heart failure, heart attack, angina, Raynaud's syndrome, loss of taste, loss of appetite, weight loss, constipation, peptic ulcer, jaundice, tiredness, dry mouth, diseases of the lymph system.

Enalapril only: Decreased blood hemoglobin, excessive perspiration, loss of consciousness, indigestion, elevated liver enzymes, nervousness, drowsiness, muscle cramps, impotence, loss of strength.

Warnings: Because of potential fall in blood pressure,

drug therapy should be under close medical supervision. Do not stop taking without doctor's orders. Use with caution by people with poor kidney function, autoimmune disease (like rheumatoid arthritis or lupus) or people on drugs affecting white blood cells or immune response. Report excessive perspiration, dehydration, vomiting, mouth sores, sore throat, fever, swelling of the hands or feet, irregular heartbeat, chest pains, water retention, skin rash, changes in taste, difficulty in breathing, diarrhea, or any signs of infection to doctor immediately. Heart patients should avoid sudden increase in physical activity. Take captopril one hour before meals. Best to stop diuretic treatment one to two weeks before starting ACE inhibitor treatment.

Possible Interactions: Patients taking diuretics may experience severe loss of blood pressure during first 3 hours after receiving the first dose of an ACE inhibitor. Avoid over-the-counter cough, cold or allergy medications. May react with blood-vessel enlargers, nitroglycerin, or other nitrates. Other blood-pressure reducers, including beta-adrenergic blocking agents and nifedipine, will increase the effects of ACE inhibitors. Spironolactone, triamterene, amiloride or potassium supplements should be used with caution. Indomethacin or aspirin decreases the effectiveness of captopril.

Antabuse® (*Ayerst*)
  See: Disulfiram

Antidiabetic Class

Generic / Brand Names:

Acetohexamide/Dymelor®
Chlorpropamide/Diabinese®
Glipizide/Glucotrol®
Glyburide/Diabeta®, Micronase®
Tolazamide/Tolinase®
Tolbutamide/Orinase®

Intended Effects: To increase the body's production of insulin in cases of mild maturity-onset diabetes.

Side Effects: Weakness, fatigue, dizziness, loss of balance or certain blood diseases such as anemia. Hypoglycemia or low blood sugar symptoms such as: anxiety, chills, drowsiness, headache, jaundice, nausea, rapid heartbeat, tiredness, vomiting; these symptoms may disappear if the dosage is lowered.

Warnings: The concentration of this drug in the body may rise to high levels in cases of kidney disease, since the body may not metabolize or excrete it properly. Should not be used in cases of juvenile diabetes or in severe cases of maturity-onset diabetes with complications such as acidosis and coma. Should not be used before surgery, after injury or in patients who have infections. Causes birth defects in animals — avoid during first three months of pregnancy. Long time use of antidiabetics may increase the chances of heart disease, so it is advisable to attempt to control maturity-onset diabetes with a low fat, low sugar, high starch diet before resorting to antidiabetics.

Possible Interactions: Antidiabetics may interfere with anticlotting drugs. Propranolol and other beta-adrenergic blocking agents may greatly increase effectiveness and lead to low blood sugar. Other drugs including aspirin, adrenal hormones, epinephrine, oral contraceptives, initial thyroid hormone replacement and thiazide diuretics can decrease effectiveness.

Antidyskinetic Class

Generic / Brand Names:
Amantadine/Symmetrel®
Benztropine/Cogentin®
Trihexyphenidyl/Artane®

Category Of Drug: Antitremor

Intended Effects: To provide relief from symptoms of Parkinson's disease, such as rigidity, tremors, sluggish movement

Side Effects: Dry mouth, blurred vision, nausea, nervousness, vomiting, constipation, numbness of fingers, listlessness, depression, skin rash, difficult urination, bloated feeling, headache, dizziness.

Warnings: Use caution when driving or operating machinery. Avoid high temperatures or over-exertion, since this drug reduces or blocks normal perspiration. Mental confusion may occur with initial large doses. Should not be used by those with glaucoma. Causes birth defects in animals — avoid during first three months of pregnancy. Known to be present in mothers' milk — avoid drug or avoid nursing.

Possible Interactions: May increase the effectiveness of levodopa and tranquilizers. May cause serious side effects when taken with cortisone, phenothiazines, or antidepressants. Effectiveness reduced when taken with antacids or medicine for diarrhea. Over the counter cough, cold or allergy medicine may cause changes in effectiveness. Dose reduction of antitremor drugs taken together should be gradual.

Antihistamine Class

Generic / Brand Names:
Azatadine/Optimine®, Trinalin®
Brompheniramine/Dimetane®
Chlorpheniramine/Chlor-Trimeton®, Teldrin®
Clemastine/Tavist®
Cyproheptadine/Periactin®
Dexchlorpheniramine/Polaramine®
Diphenhydramine/Benadryl®
Tripelennamine/PBZ®

Intended Effects: To prevent or relieve allergic symptoms, like hives, itching, rashes, swelling and difficult breathing, to prevent motion sickness, nausea and vomiting, to induce sleep. Some antihistamine preparations may be combined with phlegm looseners.

Side Effects: Most frequent: irritation from contact lenses, sedation, sleepiness, dizziness, disturbed coordination, upset stomach, and thickening of bronchial secretions. Less frequent: skin rashes (including light-sensitive skin rashes), shock, perspiration, chills, dryness of mouth, eyes, nose and throat, low blood pressure, headache, disturbance in the rhythm of the heart, anemia and other blood disorders, fatigue, confusion, restlessness, excitation, nervousness, tremor, irritability, insomnia, euphoria, numbness in the limbs, blurred vision, double vision, loss of balance, ringing in the ears, hysteria, body aches, convulsions, reduced appetite, nausea, vomiting, diarrhea, constipation, difficult urination, early menstruation, tightness of chest, wheezing, nasal stuffiness.

Warnings: Use with caution in patients with asthma, increased pressure within the eyeball, peptic ulcer, over-active thyroid, heart and vascular disease, or high blood pressure. Not advised for infants or as treatment for asthma. Known to be present in mothers' milk – avoid drug or avoid nursing.

Possible Interactions: Should not be used with MAO inhibitor antidepressants. Sedation may increase when taken with: tranquilizers, antihistamines, antidepressants, sedatives, sleep inducers, alcohol and narcotics.

Note: Some antihistamines, such as Benadryl®, are available without prescription.

Antivert® (*Roerig*)
  See: Meclizine

Anturane® (*CIBA*)
  See: Sulfinpyrazone

Anusol-HC® (*Parke-Davis*)

Category Of Drug: Rectal Cream/Suppository

Ingredients: Hydrocortisone + Bismuth + Benzyl Benzoate + Peruvian Balsam + Zinc Oxide

Intended Effects: To relieve pain, itching and discomfort of irritated anal or rectal tissues, to help reduce swelling of rectal tissue; especially helpful when inflammation is present, since it contains hydrocortisone.

Side Effects: Irritation or infection not present before using this medication could indicate sensitivity or side effects.

Warnings: Should not be used for longer period than prescribed or on any other part of the body. Use with caution in children. Usage before proper medical diagnosis may interfere with treatment of infection.

Note: See Adrenocorticoid Class - Topical

APC + Codeine
See: Salicylate Class
See: Codeine

Note: This contains aspirin, caffeine, and codeine. It no longer contains phenacetin.

Appetite Suppressant Class

Generic / Brand Names:
Benzphetamine/Didrex®
Diethylpropion/Tenuate®
Phenmetrazine/Preludin®
Phentermine/Ionamin®, Fastin®

Intended Effects: To temporarily reduce appetite

Side Effects: Elevated blood pressure, disturbed heart rhythm, overactivity, restlessness, dizziness, insomnia, euphoria, tremor, headache, psychosis, dryness of the mouth, unpleasant tastes, diarrhea, constipation, upset stomach, skin rash, changes in sex drive, impotence.

Warnings: Drugs in this class are similar to amphetamines which are addictive; tolerance may develop in a few weeks leading to increasing dosages to maintain effect. Overdoses may cause psychotic states with aggressiveness, hallucinations, and panic. Should not be taken in cases of heart disease or diseases of the blood vessels, high blood pressure, over-active thyroid, glaucoma, agitation, or patients with a history of drug abuse. Appetite suppressants should not be taken for more than a few weeks or dependence or addiction may result. Should be avoided in cases of high blood pressure.

Possible Interactions: May decrease the action of blood-pressure reducers. May increase blood pressure dangerously when taken with MAO inhibitor antidepressants. May interact with some alcoholic drinks, chocolate and meat to cause high blood pressure. Insulin requirements in diabetics may be changed in the association of appetite suppressants and diet changes.

Apresazide® (*CIBA*)
  See: Hydralazine
  See: Thiazide Diuretic Class

Apresoline® (*CIBA*)
  See: Hydralazine

Arlidin® (*USV*)
  See: Nylidrin

56

Aristocort® (*Lederle*)
See: AdrenocorticoidClass - Systemic

Aristocort A® (*Lederle*)
See: Adrenocorticoid Class - Topical

Artane® (*Lederle*)
See: Antidyskinetic Class

Ascorbic Acid (Vitamin C)

Category Of Drug: Vitamin Supplement

Intended Effects: To prevent and treat scurvy, maintain an acid urine, treat some types of anemia.

Side Effects: With large doses: diarrhea and hemolytic anemia may occur. Can cause sickle cell anemia crisis in those patients who have this disease.

Warnings: Persons taking any sulfa drug should avoid large doses of vitamin C. Pregnant and nursing women should avoid large doses — doses of several thousand milligrams per day may cause miscarriages during early pregnancy. Sodium ascorbate is the principal ingredient in some oral vitamin C preparations, therefore people on a low-sodium diet should take vitamin C only under physician's guidance. People taking large doses of vitamin C may have altered test results for urine sugar or fecal blood under certain testing situations.

Possible Interactions: Large doses may increase the effects of barbiturates, iron, sulfa drugs, aspirin. In large doses vitamin C may decrease the effects of quinidine, atropine and anticlotting drugs. If taken at the same time, vitamin C may decrease the effects of mineral oil, barbiturates, aspirin and sulfa drugs.

Note: If any allergic reaction is noted to this acid form of vitamin C, check with your doctor about trying the non-acid form: calcium ascorbate.

Ascriptin® (*Rorer*)
See· Salicylate Class

Asendin® (*Lederle*)
See: Amoxapine

Aspirin
See: Salicylate Class

Atarax® (*Roerig*)
See: Hydroxyzine

Ativan® (*Wyeth*)
See: Benzodiazepine Class

Atromid-S® (*Ayerst*)
See: Clofibrate

Augmentin® (*Beecham*)

Category Of Drug: Antibiotic

Ingredients: Amoxicillin + Clavulanate Potassium

Intended Effects: To combat infections caused by certain organisms.

Side Effects: Most frequent: diarrhea, loose stools, nausea, skin rashes, itchiness, vomiting, pain and inflammation of the vagina. Less frequent: headache, passing gas, stomach inflammation, loss of appetite, upset stomach, inflammation of the tongue, black tongue, inflammation of the colon, unusual bruising or bleeding, anemia or other blood disorders. Rare: anaphylactic shock.

Warnings: Should not be taken by anyone with a history of sensitivity to either penicillin or cephalosporin antibiotics, or by people with mononucleosis. Should be taken with caution by people who have a history of other allergic reactions. May cause false positive glucose test results. May be present in mothers' milk — avoid drug or avoid nursing. The different strength tablets contain different proportions of clavulanate to amoxicillin — so two lower strength tablets cannot be substituted for one higher strength tablet.

Possible Interactions: Augmentin® should not bᵤ used with Antabuse® (Disulfiram). Probenecid increases its effects. May cause a rash when taken with allopurinol. Other antibiotics may decrease the effectiveness of penicillins or react unfavorably with them.

Note: See Penicillin Class

Auralgan® Otic (*Ayerst*)

Category Of Drug: Decongestant, Pain Reliever

Ingredients: Antipyrine + Benzocaine + Dehydrated Glycerin.

Intended Effects: Applied in the ear canal, to relieve-pressure, reduce inflammation and congestion, and reduce pain and discomfort in acute otitis media (middle ear infection). To be used with an antibiotic to treat the infection.

Side Effects: Signs of local irritation such as burning or itching may occur.

Warnings: Not for treatment of perforated eardrum. Notify physician if burning or itching occurs. Do not use if there is a discharge from the ear.

Auranofin

Brand Name: Ridaura®

Category Of Drug: Oral gold, Anti-arthritic

Intended Effects: To treat active rheumatoid arthritis that has not responded to treatment with NSAIDs (nonsteroidal anti-inflammatory drugs), such as aspirin.

Side Effects: Most frequent (more than 10%): diarrhea, loose stools, abdominal pain or cramps, nausea, vomiting, rash, itching, inflamed stomach. Frequent (3-9%): loss of appetite, passing gas, indigestion, pink eye, protein in the urine. Less frequent (1-3%): constipation, hair loss, blood in the urine, skin rash, inflammation of the tongue, anemia and other blood disorders. Infrequent (less than 1%): stomach bleeding, fever, difficulty in swallowing, dark stools containing blood, inflammation of the colon, metallic taste, swollen and bleeding gums, jaundice, inflammation of the lungs.

Warnings: It may take three to four months or longer before the effects of auranofin can be felt. Take as prescribed. Notify physician if: diarrhea lasts four days or more; if a rash, itchiness or mouth sores develop; or if any unusual bleeding or bruising, like bleeding gums, develop. Should not be used by people with inflammation of the colon, scar tissue on the heart, or severe blood disorders. Should be used with caution in people with kidney disease, skin rash, inflammatory bowel disease, history of bone marrow depression or blood disorders. Gold-induced skin rash may be aggravated by exposure to sunlight. Not recommended for use in children. Causes birth defects in animals — avoid during pregnancy. Known to be present in mothers' milk — avoid drug or avoid nursing.

Possible Interactions: Auranofin may increase the effect of phenytoin. The safety of using auranofin with other arthritis drug treatments, including injectable gold, hydroxychloroquine, penicillamine, immunosuppres- sive drugs or high doses of corticosteroids, has not been established.

AVC® Cream (*Merrell Dow*)

Category Of Drug: Anti-infective

Ingredients: Sulfanilamide + Aminacrine + Allantoin + Lactose + Propylene Glycol + Stearic Acid + Diglycol Stearate + Trolamine + Lactic Acid

See: Sulfonamide Class - Topical

Azatadine
See: Antihistamine Class

Azo Gantanol® (*Roche*)

Category Of Drug: Anti-infective

Ingredients: Sulfamethoxazole + Phenazopyridine

See: Sulfonamide Class - Systemic
See: Phenazopyridine

Azo Gantrisin® (*Roche*)

Category Of Drug: Anti-infective

Ingredients: Sulfamethoxazole + Phenazopyridine

See: Sulfonamide Class - Systemic
See: Phenazopyridine

Azulfidine® (*Pharmacia*)
See: Sulfonamide Class - Systemic

Bacampicillin
See: Penicillin Class

Bactrim® (*Roche*)
See: Sulfonamide Class-Systemic

Barbiturate Class

Generic / Brand Names:
Butalbital
Butabarbital/Butisol Sodium®
Mephobarbital/Mebaral®
Pentobarbital/Nembutal®
Phenobarbital
Secobarbital/Seconal®

Category Of Drug: Sedative, Anticonvulsant, Sleeping Aid

Intended Effects: The long-acting forms provide relief of anxiety or tension. The short-term types are taken at bedtime to cause sleep or in continuous, regularly scheduled doses, to prevent epileptic seizures.

Side Effects: Breathing difficulties, skin rash, runny nose, watery eyes, scratchy throat, drowsiness, lack of energy, nausea, vomiting, diarrhea, anemia, jaundice, dizziness, liver problems, excitement, depression, confusion, headache.

Warnings: Should not be taken by people who have had liver problems or serious respiratory disorders. Should not be taken by people who have had drug addiction problems, since ordinary doses may not be effective and may lead to further addiction problems. Should be used with caution by those driving or operating machinery. Causes birth defects in animals — do not use during first three months of pregnancy. Known to be present in mothers' milk — avoid drug or avoid nursing. In small doses, may actually increase sensations of pain. Prolonged use may result in addictive dependence; sudden withdrawal in such cases may prove fatal. Emotional disturbances may be increased.

Possible Interactions: Sedation may increase when taken with: tranquilizers, antihistamines, antidepressants, sedatives, sleep inducers, alcohol and narcotics. Barbiturates may decrease the effectiveness of other medications such as anticlotting drugs or adrenal hormones.

Beclomethasone

Brand Name: Vanceril®

Category Of Drug: Adrenal Hormone

Intended Effects: Only for use in cases of severe asthma which cannot be controlled by bronchial tube relaxers and other non-adrenocorticoid medications.

Side Effects: Death from adrenal insufficiency; dry mouth, fungus infections of the mouth, throat and larynx. Rinsing the mouth and gargling after each use of this drug may help reduce development of fungal mouth and throat infections.

Warnings: Should not be used in cases of non-asthmatic bronchitis or in cases of asthma which can be controlled by non-corticosteroid medications. Should not be used by people who require non-inhalation corticosteroid treatment. Deaths due to adrenal insufficiency have occurred in asthmatic patients during and after changing from other adrenocorticoid drugs to this aerosol. The manufacturer recommends a period of several months of gradual withdrawal from oral adrenocorticoid therapy for the body's hormone system to recover while using Vanceril® in inhalation therapy. The manufacturer further recommends that patients should be instructed to resume other adrenocorticoid medication in large doses immediately after a severe asthmatic attack. Animal studies suggest that high doses of this aerosol drug or long term use can stop growth and sexual maturation. In addition, a high incidence of convulsions and incoordinated movements were attributed to the inhalation of excessive amounts of the fluorocarbon propellent in this aerosol. Causes birth defects in animals — avoid during first three months of pregnancy.

Possible Interactions: Oral or inhaled bronchial-tube relaxers may increase Vanceril® effects.

Beepen VK® *(Beecham Labs)*
See: Penicillin Class

Bellergal-S® *(Sandoz)*

Category Of Drug: Tranquilizer

Ingredients: Phenobarbital + Ergotamine + Belladonna

Intended Effects: To treat disorders characterized by nervous tension such as menopausal disorders, nervous stomach, certain heart problems, premenstrual tension, recurrent throbbing headache.

Side Effects: Dry mouth, blurred vision, flushing. Rare: drowsiness.

Warnings: Should be avoided by people with coronary heart disease, high blood pressure, impaired kidney function or glaucoma. Special caution is advised if this drug is used by patients with bronchial asthma. Since it contains a barbiturate, this drug may be habit-forming. People sensitive to ergot may develop heart problems. Causes birth defects in animals — avoid during first three months of pregnancy. Known to be present in mothers' milk — avoid drug or avoid nursing.

Possible Interactions: Interacts with anticlotting drugs and phenytoin. Sedation may increase when taken with: tranquilizers, antihistamines, antidepressants, sleep inducers, sedatives, alcohol, narcotics and diuretics.

Note: See Barbiturate Class

Benadryl® (*Parke-Davis*)
  See: Antihistamine Class

Note: No Rx prescription required

Benemid® (*Merck Sharp & Dohme*)
  See: Probenecid

Bentyl® (*Merrell Dow*)
  See: Dicyclomine

Bentyl® + Phenobarbital (*Merrell Dow*)
See: Barbiturate Class
See: Dicyclomine

Benylin® Cough Syrup (*Parke-Davis*)
See: Antihistamine Class

Note: No Rx prescription required

Benzodiazepine Class

Generic / Brand Names:
  Alprazolam/Xanax®
  Chlordiazepoxide/Librium®
  Clorazepate/Tranxene®
  Diazepam/Valium®
  Flurazepam/Dalmane®
  Lorazepam/Ativan®
  Oxazepam/Serax®
  Prazepam/Centrax®
  Triazolam/Halcion®

Category Of Drug: Tranquilizer

Intended Effects: To relieve short-term anxiety caused by trauma or stress, to reduce agitation and delirium in alcohol withdrawal, to relieve muscle spasms, to induce sleep.

Side Effects: Frequent: drowsiness, fatigue, lack of muscle coordination. Less frequent: confusion, constipation, depression, double vision, headache, low blood pressure,

67

jaundice, changes in sex-drive, nausea, changes in salivation, skin rash, slurred speech, tremor, urinary difficulties, loss of balance, blurred vision, excitation, anxiety, hallucinations, increased muscle spasms, insomnia, rage, sleep disturbances.

Warnings: May be physically and psychologically habit-forming. Abrupt discontinuation after taking high doses for a long period of time can cause convulsions, tremor, abdominal and muscle cramps, vomiting and sweating; gradual withdrawal is recommended after extensive use. Use should be avoided by small children, by people with a known sensitivity to minor tranquilizers, and by people with acute narrow-angle glaucoma.

Possible Interactions: Sedation may increase when taken with: tranquilizers, antihistamines, antidepressants, sedatives, sleep inducers, alcohol and narcotics. The action of high blood pressure reducers may be increased The effectiveness of anticonvulsants may be decreased. Disulfiram and Tagamet® (cimetidine) may cause increased effects.

Benzphetamine
See: Appetite Suppressant Class

Benztropine
See: Antidyskinetic Class

Berocca® (*Roche*)

Category Of Drug: Vitamin Supplement

Ingredients: Vitamin C (ascorbic acid) B-complex (B1, B2, B6, B12, Niacinamide, Calcium, Pantothenate, Folic acid)

Intended Effects: For nutritional supplement. The ascorbic acid aids in tissue repair and bone protein formation. For nutritional support as in pregnancy, burn treatment, over active thyroid production, alcoholism, diabetes, and extensive aspirin treatment.

Side Effects: Rare: diarrhea, flushing, headache, nausea, vomiting, stomach cramps and abdominal pain.

Warnings: Not for treatment of anemias. Use with caution in people with gout.

Possible Interactions: Increases effect of methenamine

Note: See Ascorbic Acid

Berocca-C® (*Roche*)
See: Berocca®
See: Ascorbic Acid

Note: A vitamin supplement given by injection.

Beta-Adrenergic Blocking Agent Class

Generic / Brand Names:
Acebutolol/Sectral®
Atenolol/Tenormin®
Metoprolol/Lopressor®

Nadolol/Corgard®
Pindolol/Visken®
Propranolol/Inderal®
Timolol/Blocadren®, Timolide®

Category Of Drug: Blood-Pressure Reducer

Intended Effects: To reduce blood pressure, to slow and strengthen heartbeat, to regulate irregular heartbeat, to reduce oxygen requirements of the heart, to reduce the chances of stroke and other complications of high blood pressure, to reduce the rate of heart attacks caused by atherosclerosis, to prevent migraine headaches, to reduce the pain of angina pectoris. Recent studies prove the effectiveness of beta-blockers in reducing fatalities associated with high blood pressure and fatalities in post-heart-attack patients.

Side Effects: Frequent: numbness in hands, arms or feet, faintness upon rising, depression, tiredness, dizziness, slow pulse, diarrhea, cold hands or feet, dryness of mouth and nausea. Less frequent: hallucinations, headache, sleeping problems, constipation, difficulty in breathing and disorientation.

Warnings: Close monitoring of patient by physician is necessary to determine if the desired effects are being produced. Angina patients should not discontinue suddenly. Causes birth defects in animals — avoid during the first three months of pregnancy. Known to be present in mothers' milk — avoid drug or avoid nursing. May interfere with heart activity during major surgery. May interfere with treatment of overactive thyroid, low blood sugar, diabetes, kidney or liver disease. May seriously increase breathing difficulty in cases of asthma or hay fever. May cause the vagus nerve to be oversensitive and cause a dangerously low heart rate.

70

Possible Interactions: Sedation may increase when taken with: tranquilizers, antihistamines, antidepressants, sedatives, sleep inducers, alcohol, narcotics, reserpine, and phenytoin. May decrease the effects of anti-inflammatory drugs and antihistamines. May lower blood pressure excessively if alcohol is consumed. May increase the properties of antidiabetic drugs and insulin.

Beta-Blockers
See: Beta-Adrenergic Blocking Agent Class

Betamethasone
See: Adrenocorticoid Class-Systemic or Topical

Bethanechol

Brand Name: Urecholine®

Category Of Drug: Nervous-System Regulator

Intended Effects: To treat acute urinary retention caused by poor function of the nervous system or following surgery or childbirth.

Side Effects: Abdominal discomfort, salivation, flushing of the skin, sweating. With large doses: "unwell" or "achy" feeling, headache, sensation of heat about the face, flushing, diarrhea, nausea, belching, abdominal cramps, asthmatic attacks, drop in blood pressure, shock or heart attack.

Warnings: Not for those with overactive thyroid, peptic ulcer, bronchial asthma, very slow heart rate, low or unstable blood pressure, coronary artery disease, epilepsy or parkinsonism. Should not be used with weak stomach, intestine or bladder walls, in cases of bladder or bladder neck obstruction, or following recent urinary bladder surgery, or when stomach or intestinal cramps, ulcers or inflammation are present.

Possible Interactions: A critical fall in blood pressure, usually preceeded by severe abdominal symptoms, may occur if this drug is given to patients receiving other nervous system regulators or certain blood pressure reducers.

Bisacodyl
  See: Laxative-Stimulant Class

Bitolterol Mesylate

Brand Name: Tornalate® Metered Dose Inhaler

Category Of Drug: Bronchial-Tube Relaxer

Intended Effects: To relieve difficult breathing associated with bronchial asthma and reversible bronchospasm.

Side Effects: Tremors, nervousness, throat irritation, coughing, headache, dizziness, lightheadedness, nausea, awareness of heartbeat, chest discomfort, increased heart rate, changes in blood pressure, insomnia, restlessness, chest tightness, difficult breathing, narrowing of air passages in the lungs.

Warnings: Should be used with caution by people with heart disease, high blood pressure, overactive thyroid, diabetes, irregular heartbeat, or convulsive disorders.

Possible Interactions: Do not use with other aerosol bronchial-tube relaxers because they may have additive effects.

Bleph®-10 Liquifilm® (*Allergan*)

Category Of Drug: Anti-infective

Ingredients: Sulfacetamide Sodium + Thimerosal + Polyvinyl Alcohol + Polysorbate 80 + Sodium Thiosulfate + Potassium Phosphate Monobasic + Edetate Disodium + Sodium Phosphate Dibasic + Anhydrous + Hydrochloric Acid + Purified Water.

Intended Effects: To treat conjunctivitis (pinkeye), corneal ulcer and superficial eye infections.

Side Effects: Eye irritation in people sensitive to sulfa drugs.

Warnings: Do not use if solution is dark brown. Protect from light and high heat. May promote fungus infections.

Possible Interactions: Do not use with medicine containing silver.

Blephamide® (*Allergan*)

Category Of Drug: Anti-inflammatory, Anti-infective

Ingredients: Sulfacetamide Sodium + Prednisolone Acetate

Intended Effects: To treat bacterial infections of the eye, to treat injury to the cornea of the eye caused by chemicals, radiation, burns or wounds.

Side Effects: Fungus infections after long-term use, increased allergic reactions, raised intra-eye pressure. Prolonged use may cause glaucoma and increase the chance of eye infections.

Warnings: May hinder the body's defenses against infection. People allergic to sulfa drugs or thiazide diuretics may also be allergic to this drug. If the ingredients in this drug are taken internally, as in other preparations, they are known to cause birth defects in animals and to be present in mothers' milk.

Possible Interactions: Aminobenzoic acid eye medicine may cause decreased effects. Do not take with medicine containing silver.

Blocadren® (*Merck Sharp & Dohme*)
See: Beta-Adrenergic Blocking Agent Class

Brethine® (*Geigy*)
See: Terbutaline

Brevicon® (*Syntex*)

See: Estrogen + Progestin   Class

Brompheniramine
See: Antihistamine Class

Bronkometer® (*Breon*)
See: Isoetharine

Bronkosol® (*Breon*)
See: Isoetharine

Buffered Aspirin
See: Salicylate Class

BuSpar® (*Mead Johnson*)
See: Buspirone

Buspirone

Brand Name: BuSpar®

Category Of Drug: Anti-anxiety

Intended Effects: To manage anxiety disorders; for short-term relief of the symptoms of anxiety.

Side Effects: Most frequent: dizziness, nausea,

nervousness, headache, lightheadedness, excitement, depression, drowsiness, insomnia, fatigue, weakness, sedation, tingling sensations, diarrhea, chest pain, dream disturbances, ringing in the ears, sore throat, nasal congestion. Infrequent: lack of concentration, anger, confusion, blurred vision, constipation, vomiting, numbness, incoordination, tremors, skin rash, sweating, fainting, low blood pressure, high blood pressure, intolerance to noise, a feeling of wellbeing, fearfulness, loss of interest, seizures, hallucinations, suicidal ideas, redness and itching of the eyes, altered taste, altered smell, pink eye, flatulence, loss of appetite, increased appetite, salivation, irritable colon, bleeding from the rectum, increased urination, reduced urination, difficult urination, joint pain, menstrual irregularities, menstrual spotting, muscle cramps, muscle spasm, stiff muscles, involuntary movements, slowed reaction time, hyperventilation, shortness of breath, chest congestion, changes in sex drive, itching, bruising, dry skin, swelling in the face, blisters, weight gain, weight loss, fever, "unwell" feeling, fluid retention, swelling.

Warnings: May be effective for only short-term (three to four weeks) treatment. Use caution while driving or operating machinery if drowsiness occurs. Since buspirone is not

a benzodiazepine, people taking benzodiazepines prior to buspirone should be eased off of their old drug before starting buspirone treatment. Should not be used by people with poor kidney or liver function. Known to be present in mothers' milk– avoid drug or avoid nursing. May take several days before buspirone is effective.

Possible Interactions: Trazodone (Desyrel®) and BuSpar® may cause changes in liver function when taken together. Sedation may increase when taken with: tranquilizers, antihistamines, antidepressants, sedatives, sleep inducers, alcohol or narcotics. Because of lack of experience, buspirone and other drugs that affect the central nervous system should only be used together with extreme caution. May react with Digoxin (Lanoxin®) when taken together.

Butabarbital
See: Barbiturate Class

Butazolidin® (*Geigy*)
See: Phenylbutazone

Butisol Sodium® (*Wallace*)
See: Barbiturate Class

Cafergot® (*Sandoz*)

Category Of Drug: Blood-Vessel Reducer

Ingredients: Ergotamine tartrate + Caffeine

Intended Effects: To relieve and prevent certain headaches, like migraines; to relieve drowsiness.

Side Effects: Nervousness, insomnia, weak pulse, muscle pains, weakness, nausea, vomiting, itching.

Warnings: Overdoses may cause fatal poisoning. Causes abortion — do not use during pregnancy! Known to be present in mothers' milk — avoid drug or avoid nursing. Prolonged use of high doses may cause tolerance and psychological dependence. Avoid possible overdose by limiting caffeine beverages. Not for patients with active stomach ulcer or severe heart disease. With extended use can aggravate fibrocystic breast disease.

Possible Interactions: Sedation may increase when taken with: tranquilizers, antihistamines, antidepressants, sedatives, sleep inducers, alcohol and narcotics. Can increase the effects of thyroid preparations and amphetamines. Interacts with MAO inhibitors. Meprobamate and isoniazid may increase the effects of this drug.

Calan® (*Searle*)
  See: Calcium Channel Inhibitor Class

Calcium Channel Inhibitor Class

Generic / Brand Names:
  Diltiazem/Cardizem®
  Nifedipine/Procardia®

  Verapamil/Calan®, Isoptin®
Category Of Drug: Anti-angina, Blood-Vessel Enlarger

Intended Effects: To relieve pain associated with hardening of the coronary arteries (angina).

Side Effects: Dizziness, lightheadedness, flushing, hot feeling, headache, weakness, nausea, heartburn, cramps, tremors, fluid retention, nervousness, pounding heart beat, mood changes, wheezing, congestion, sore throat, breathlessness.

Warnings: Causes birth defects in animals; may harm fetus. Avoid or use cautiously during pregnancy.

Possible Interactions: Don't withdraw suddenly from beta blockers before or during therapy. Taking beta blockers at the same time is usually well tolerated, but many cause heart failure in people with aorta problems, who are also taking beta blockers.

Capoten® (*Squibb*)
See: Angiotensin Converting Enzyme (ACE) Inhibitor Class

Captopril
See: Angiotensin Converting Enzyme Inhibitor Class

Carafate® (*Marion*)
See: Sucralfate

Carbamazepine

Brand Name: Tegretol®

Category Of Drug: Anticonvulsant, Pain-Reliever

Intended Effects: To treat epilepsy when other drugs have failed. To treat trigeminal neuralgia.

Side Effects: Most frequently during initial stages of treatment: dizziness, drowsiness, unsteadiness, nausea, vomiting. Less frequent: aplastic anemia, low white blood cell count, liver function abnormalities, urinary difficulties, confusion (especially in the elderly), headache, fatigue, blurred vision, speech disturbances, involuntary movements, skin rash, itching, hives, exaggerated sunburn, dryness of mouth and throat, loss of appetite, congestive heart failure, changes in blood pressure, fluid retention, aching of muscles and joints, leg cramps. Rare: heart attacks, strokes, phlebitis.

Warnings: Not for people with history of bone marrow depression, active liver disease or known sensitivity to any of the tricyclic antidepressants. Causes birth defects in animals — avoid during first three months of pregnancy. Known to be present in mothers' milk — avoid drug or avoid nursing. Drive or operate machinery with caution. Should be used with caution by people with high blood pressure, heart disease, history of serious mental or emotional disorders, glaucoma.

Possible Interactions: This drug may increase the sedative effects of alcohol. Tricyclic antidepressants may interact with this drug. Not recommended for people taking MAO

inhibitors unless 14 days have elapsed.

Carbenicillin
See: Penicillin Class

Carbinoxamine
See: Antihistamine Class

Cardizem® (*Marion*)
   See: Calcium Channel Inhibitor Class

Carisoprodol

Brand Name: Soma®

Category Of Drug: Muscle Relaxant

Intended Effects: To relieve discomfort caused by spasms of voluntary muscles.

Side Effects: Weakness, lethargy, drowsiness, dizziness, lightheadedness, tremor, agitation, irritability, headache, mental depression, insomnia, skin rash, indigestion, nausea, rapid heartbeat. Rare: reaction to the first dose may include: extreme weakness, dizziness, temporary loss of vision, slurred speech, confusion, temporary paralysis of legs and arms — these symptoms usually lessen over several hours.

Warnings: Known to be present in mothers' milk — avoid drug or avoid nursing. Not for children under the age of 12. If used in large doses for a long period of time, psychological and physical dependence can result. Should be used with caution by people with poor kidney or liver function. Not for people with acute intermittent porphyria. People allergic to meprobamate, mebutamate or tybamate may also be allergic to this drug.

Possible Interactions: Sedation may increase when taken with: tranquilizers, antihistamines, antidepressants, sedatives, sleep inducers, alcohol and narcotics.

Catapres® (*Boehringer*)
See: Clonidine

Ceclor® (*Lilly*)
See: Cephalosporin Class

Cefaclor
See: Cephalosporin Class

Cefadroxil
See: Cephalosporin Class

Centrax® (*Parke-Davis*)
See: Benzodiazepine Class

Cephalexin
See: Cephalosporin Class

Cephalosporin Class

Generic / Brand Names:
Cefaclor/Ceclor®
Cefadroxil/Duricef®
Cephalexin/Keflex®
Cephradine/Velosef®

Category Of Drug: Antibiotic

Intended Effects: To combat infections caused by certain bacteria: on the skin, in the middle ear, respiratory tract or urinary tract.

Side Effects: Diarrhea, nausea, vomiting, upset stomach, abdominal pain, infection of the colon, rashes, fluid congestion around the heart, genital and anal fungus infections, dizziness, fatigue and headache.

Warnings: Should be avoided by people who are allergic to penicillin or cephalosporin products. Should be used with caution by people with poor kidney function. Known to be present in mothers' milk — avoid drug or avoid nursing Most effective when taken one hour before or two hours after eating. May cause false readings in diabetics using tablets for sugar tests.

Possible Interactions: The effectiveness of anticlotting drugs increases when taken with cephalosporins. Probenecid may increase the levels of cephalosporins in the blood, since it may interfere with normal elimination.

Cephradine
See: Cephalosporin Class

Chloral Hydrate

Brand Name: Noctec®

Category Of Drug: Sleeping Aid

Intended Effects: To relieve mild anxiety or tension and insomnia.

Side Effects: Upset stomach, faintness upon rising, weakness, unsteadiness, drowsiness, skin rashes, nightmares, headache, nausea.

Warnings: Should be taken with a full glass of liquid. Known to be present in mothers' milk — avoid drug or avoid nursing. May be habit-forming. Do not stop taking suddenly. Not for patients with stomach inflammation, severe kidney or liver problems. Drive or use hazardous machinery with caution.

Possible Interactions: Chloral hydrate may reduce effectiveness of some anticlotting drugs. Sedation may increase when taken with: tranquilizers, antihistamines, antidepressants, sedatives, sleep inducers, alcohol and narcotics, even to the point of unconsciousness.

Chloramphenicol

Brand Name: Chloroptic®

Category Of Drug: Antibiotic

Intended Effects: To treat superficial eye infections.

Side Effects: Burning or stinging, diarrhea, development of a second infection, skin rash, swelling of face or limbs, fever, nausea, vomiting, irritation of mouth or tongue.

Warnings: Consult physician if sore throat, fever pale skin, unusual bleeding, bruising, tiredness or weakness occur while taking this drug or after treatment has ended. May cause birth defects in animals — avoid during first three months of pregnancy. Known to be present in mothers' milk — avoid drug or avoid nursing.

Possible Interactions: This drug may increase the effects of certain antidiabetic drugs, phenytoin and dicumarol. May decrease the effects of penicillin and cyclophosphamide. When taken with alcohol, may cause nausea and other side effects.

Note: Side effects are less common when this drug is applied topically.

Chlordiazepoxide
See: Benzodiazepine Class

Chloroptic® (*Allergan*)
See: Chloramphenicol

Chlorothiazide
See: Thiazide Diuretic Class

Chlorpheniramine
See: Antihistamine Class

Chlorpromazine
See: Phenothiazine Class

Chlorpropamide
See: Antidiabetic Class

Chlorthalidone
See: Thiazide Diuretic Class

Chlor-Trimeton® (*Schering*)
See: Antihistamine   Class

Note: No Rx prescription required

Choledyl® (*Parke-Davis*)
See: Xanthine Class

Cimetidine

Brand Name: Tagamet®

Category Of Drug: Stomach Acid Secretion Inhibitor

Intended Effects: To treat stomach ulcer and duodenal ulcer pain by shutting off the flow of stomach acid and allowing ulcers to heal, to prevent the recurrence of ulcers when given at a lower dosage by restricting the secretion of acid. Highly effective in treating duodenal ulcers; probably effective in treating stomach ulcers as well.

Side Effects: Diarrhea, muscle pain, dizziness, rash, headache, tremor, enlargement of breasts, heart irregularities, low blood pressure.

Warnings: A slight feminizing effect may occur after prolonged treatment. Do not discontinue abruptly.

Possible Interactions: The activity of anticlotting drugs may be increased. Benzodiazepines, such as the tranquilizers Valium® and Librium®, may be eliminated from the body at higher rates when cimetidine is taken at the same time. Caffeine and alcoholic beverages may reduce the effectiveness of this drug and delay ulcer healing.

Clemastine
   See: Antihistamine Class

Cleocin™ (*Upjohn*)
   See: Clindamycin

Cleocin T™ (*Upjohn*)
   See: Clindamycin

Clindamycin

Brand Names: Cleocin™, Cleocin T™

Category Of Drug: Antibiotic

Intended Effects: To treat infections.

Side Effects: Persistent and troublesome diarrhea,

abdominal pain, dryness, fatigue, headache, oily skin, sore throat, eye irritation, frequent urination. Development of second infection.

Warnings: Consult physician at once if diarrhea and severe stomach cramps develop; may indicate potentially serious colitis condition. Known to be present in mothers' milk — avoid drug or avoid nursing. Contains an alcohol base which will cause irritation and burning of the eyes, cuts, or mucous membranes — if contact is made bathe with large amounts of cool tap water. Avoid if allergic to lincomycin. Not recommended for patients with history of ulcerative colitis.

Possible Interactions: Antidiarrhea medications may decrease its effects.

Note: Side effects are less common when clindamycin is applied topically.

Clinoril® *(Merck Sharp & Dohme)*
  See: Sulindac

Clofibrate

Brand Name: Atromid-S®

Category Of Drug: Blood-Fat Reducer

Intended Effects: To reduce high blood levels of cholesterol and triglycerides.

Side Effects: Most frequent: nausea. Less frequent: weight gain, allergic skin reactions, vomiting, fatigue, drowsiness, headache, flu-like symptoms, impotence, abnormal liver function, anemia.

Warnings: Long term use of this drug advised only under physician's orders because of possibility of increase in serious disorders or diseases. Avoid while nursing. This drug should be discontinued gradually after 3 months if no significant improvement in blood cholesterol and/or triglycerides has occurred. May harm fetus; strict birth control methods should be practiced before, after and while taking this drug.

Possible Interactions: Anticlotting drugs may cause increased effects.

Clomid® (*Merrell Dow*)
  See: Clomiphene

Clomiphene

Brand Name: Clomid®

Category Of Drug: Fertility Aid

Intended Effects: To treat infertility in women and men. (Promotes ovulation in two thirds of women who do not ovulate).

Side Effects: Hot flashes, vision difficulties, headache, dizziness.

Warnings: Not recommended for patients with impaired

kidney function, vaginal bleeding or ovarian cysts. Pregnant women should avoid this drug since birth defects may result. Use of this drug may increase chances of multiple pregnancies but not as much as with certain other drugs. Patients taking clomiphene should follow drug schedule carefully. Overdoses may cause ovaries to rupture. Stomach or pelvic pain and bloating may indicate cyst formation or ovary enlargement — patient should notify physician if these symptoms occur.

Clonidine

Brand Name: Catapres®

Category Of Drug: Blood-Pressure Reducer

Intended Effects: To lower high blood pressure.

Side Effects: Dry mouth, drowsiness, sedation, constipation, dizziness, headache, fatigue, nausea, vomiting, liver problems, weight gain, blood sugar problems, heart problems, vivid dreams, sleeplessness, nervousness, anxiety, depression, rash, itching, thinning of hair, impotence, difficult urination, burning or itching eyes.

Warnings: May cause birth defects in animals — avoid during first three months of pregnancy. Should be discontinued gradually, not suddenly. Caution should be used when driving or operating machinery. Should be used with caution in patients having severe heart or kidney problems. Patients using this drug for prolonged periods should have regular eye exams.

Possible Interactions: Use cautiously with alcohol.

Sedation may increase when taken with: tranquilizers, anti-histamines, sedatives, sleep inducers, alcohol and narcotics. Antidepressants may decrease its action.

Clorazepate
See: Benzodiazepine Class

Clotrimazole - Topical

Brand Names: Gyne-Lotrimin®, Lotrimin®

Category Of Drug: Antifungus

Intended Effects: To treat yeast-like fungus infections in the vagina or on the skin.

Side Effects: When used in the vagina: burning, irritation, cystitis. When used on the skin: hives, blistering, stinging, redness of the skin, general irritation.

Warnings: Consult physician if irritation or sensitivity occurs. Do not use near the eyes. If symptoms do not respond to this drug, condition may be caused by different micro-organisms which are not susceptible to it, and other therapy should be tried.

Cloxacillin
See: Penicillin Class

Codeine

Category Of Drug: Pain Reliever, Narcotic, Anticough

Intended Effects: To reduce pain, to prevent coughing spasms, to supplement the action of other drugs.

Side Effects: Drowsiness, constipation, lightheadedness, dizziness, fainting, shortness of breath, slowed heartbeat, excitement, difficult urination, loss of appetite, tiredness, flushing of face and neck.

Warnings: Drugs containing codeine can be habit forming, and tolerance may develop, which leads to increased use. Causes birth defects in animals — avoid during first three months of pregnancy. Known to be present in mothers' milk – avoid drug or avoid nursing.

Possible Interactions: Sedation may increase when taken with: tranquilizers, antihistamines, antidepressants, sedatives, sleep inducers, alcohol, narcotics — use cautiously with phenytoin, chloramphenicol or alcohol.

Cogentin® (*Merck Sharp & Dohme*)
  See: Antidyskinetic Class

Colace® (*Mead Johnson*)
  See: Laxative-Emollient   Class

ColBenemid® (*Merck Sharp & Dohme*)
  See: Colchicine
  See: Probenecid

Colchicine

Category Of Drug: Anti-gout

Intended Effects: To relieve pain, swelling and inflammation of gout. To reduce further attacks of gout.

Side Effects: Nausea, vomiting, diarrhea, stomach cramps, rash, fever, hives. With long-term use: bloody diarrhea, decreased ability of bone marrow to produce blood cells, anemia, numbness in limbs, liver damage.

Warnings: Causes birth defects in animals — avoid during first three months of pregnancy. Should be used with caution by the elderly, infirm, or patients with heart disease, impaired kidney or liver function, peptic ulcer or ulcerative colitis. May cause serious bleeding problems for patients with stomach or intestinal ulcers or active ulcerative colitis. Notify physician if severe diarrhea develops.

Possible Interactions: Sedation may increase when taken with: tranquilizers, antihistamines, antidepressants, sedatives, sleep inducers, alcohol and narcotics. May decrease the effects of blood-pressure reducing and anticlotting drugs.

Coly-Mycin® S Otic (*Parke-Davis*)

Category Of Drug: Antibacterial, Anti-inflammatory

Ingredients: Coly-Mycin + Neomycin + Hydrocortisone

Intended Effects: To treat bacterial infections of the outer ear canal and infections after mastoid surgery.

Side Effects: Fungus infections with prolonged treatment. Reddening of the skin, rash, itching, burning sensations.

Warnings: Should be used with caution by patients with perforated eardrum or chronic middle ear infection. Not for people with herpes simplex, fungus infections or viral infections of the ear. Do not heat this medicine above body temperature.

Possible Interactions: Allergic reactions may occur with kanamycin, paromomycin, streptomycin and gentamicin.

Combid® (*Smith Kline & French*)

Category Of Drug: Nervous-System Regulator, Tranquilizer, Antispasm.

Ingredients: Prochlorperazine + Isopropamide

Intended Effects: To treat discomfort of excessive activity and spasm of the digestive tract; to help control diarrhea, peptic ulcer and irritable bowel syndrome, to control nausea.

Side Effects: Dry mouth and throat, blurred vision, constipation, urinary problems, dizziness, headache, nausea, hives, skin rash, rapid heart beat, liver damage.

Warnings: In hot weather this drug may increase the risk of heat stroke. Use with caution in elderly patients or in people with history of jaundice or liver irregularities. Causes birth defects in animals — avoid during first three months of pregnancy. Known to be present in mothers' milk — avoid drug or avoid nursing. Not for people with glaucoma, bladder neck obstruction, bone marrow reduction, existing drug-induced depression, or severe ulcerative colitis.

Possible Interactions: May intensify and prolong action of pain relievers, antihistamines, barbiturates, alcohol and atropine. Interacts with MAO inhibitors and some glaucoma medications.

Note: See also Phenothiazine Class

Combipres® (*Boehringer*)
  See: Clonidine
  See: Thiazide Diuretic Class

Compazine® (*Smith Kline & French*)
  See: Phenothiazine Class

Co-Pyronil® 2 (*Dista*)

Category Of Drug: Antihistamine

Ingredients: Chlorpheniramine + Pseudoephedrine

Intended Effects: To relieve symptoms of hay fever, allergic headache and gastrointestinal allergy.

Side Effects: Sedation, dryness of throat, nose and mouth, dizziness, disturbed coordination, fatigue, confusion, restlessness, excitability, nervousness, insomnia, nausea, vomiting, tightness of chest, wheezing, blurred vision, nasal stuffiness, urinary problems.

Warnings: Should be used with caution in patients with history of bronchial asthma, glaucoma, high blood pressure, diabetes, heart disease, kidney disease, overactive thyroid. May cause diminished mental alertness. Drive and operate machinery with caution. May produce excitation in young children. This drug should not be used by people sensitive to any of its ingredients.

Possible Interactions: MAO inhibitors prolong the drying effects of this drug. Sedation may increase when taken with; tranquilizers, antihistamines, antidepressants, sedatives, sleep inducers, alcohol and narcotics.

Note: No Rx prescription required.

Cordran® *(Dista)*
  See: Adrenocorticoid Class-Topical

Corgard® *(Squibb)*
  See: Beta-Adrenergic Blocking Agent Class

Cortisporin® **Ointment** *(Burroughs Wellcome)*

Category Of Drug: Antibiotic, Anti-inflammatory

Ingredients: Polymyxin B + Bacitracin + Neomycin + Hydrocortisone

Intended Effects: To treat topical bacterial infections such as wounds, burns and skin grafts. To aid in treating certain eczema conditions and in healing after certain types of surgery.

Side Effects: Reddening, swelling, dry scaling and itching of treated area. Prolonged use may result in fungus growth.

Warnings: Should not be used over large areas of the body, because great absorption through the skin may cause kidney damage. Not for use on deep or puncture wounds, raw areas or serious burns unless physician recommends.

Cortisporin® Ophthalmic (*Burroughs Wellcome*)

Category Of Drug: Anti-inflammatory, Anti-infective, Anti-itching.

Ingredients: Polymyxin B + Bacitracin + Neomycin + Hydrocortisone

Intended Effects: To treat eye conditions caused by bacterial infections, or conjunctivitis, to treat superficial chemical and heat burns of the cornea.

Side Effects: Irritation, fungus infections.

Warnings: Long-term use may result in optic nerve or cataract damage. Should be avoided by people with certain fungal or viral injuries of the skin or eye, tuberculosis, or herpes simplex. Consult physician if itching, redness, swelling, rash or other symptoms of irritation occur, since this may indicate sensitivity to the drug.

Cortisporin® Otic (*Burroughs Wellcome*)

Category Of Drug: Antibiotic, Anti-itching, Anti-inflammatory, Anti-allergy

Ingredients: Polymyxin B + Neomycin + Hydrocortisone

Intended Effects: To treat bacterial infections of the outer ear canal.

Side Effects: Reddening, swelling, dry scaling. Fungus infections may result when treatment is prolonged. If medication reaches the middle ear: stinging and burning.

Warnings: Consult physician if irritation of ear occurs from this medication. Do not heat this medication above body temperature. Not for people with herpes simplex. Maximum treatment length is ten days.

Possible Interactions: May interact with other antibiotics such as kanamycin, paromomycin, or streptomycin.

Coumadin® (*Du Pont*)
See: Warfarin

Cyclacillin
See: Penicillin Class

Cyclandelate

Brand Name: Cyclospasmol®

Category Of Drug: Blood-Vessel Enlarger

Intended Effects: To promote better blood circulation for patients with hardening of the arteries, nightly leg cramps, and certain brain circulation disorders. Best results are achieved with long-term use.

Side Effects: Stomach irritation, nausea, heartburn, flushing, headache, weakness, rapid heartbeat. Many of these can be avoided by taking medicine at mealtime or with antacids.

Warnings: Should not be used by patients who are sensitive to the drug. Should be used with caution by patients with severe heart or brain artery conditions or patients with glaucoma. Prolongs bleeding time; use cautiously in people with active bleeding or bleeding tendency. Causes birth defects in animals — avoid during first three months of pregnancy.

Possible Interactions: Nicotine in tobacco may reduce this drug's ability to improve circulation.

Cyclapen-W® *(Wyeth)*
See: Penicillin Class

Cyclobenzaprine

Brand Name: Flexeril®

Category Of Drug: Muscle Relaxant

Intended Effects: To treat pain, tenderness, limitation of motion and restriction of activities caused by muscle spasms.

Side Effects: Drowsiness, dry mouth, dizziness, increased heart rate, weakness, fatigue, nausea, sweating, constipation, excessive sunburn, skin rash, disturbed concentration.

Warnings: Not for long term therapy. Drive or operate machinery with caution. Known to be present in mothers' milk — avoid drug or avoid nursing. Should be used with caution by those with urinary retention, glaucoma, increased intra-eye pressure and those taking nervous system regulators. Not for those recovering from recent heart attack, those with overactive thyroid, congestive heart failure, or those who are taking or have taken within the last 14 days MAO inhibitor antidepressants.

Possible Interactions: Convulsions may result if this drug is taken with MAO inhibitor antidepressants. May block the action of guanethidine. Sedation may increase when taken with: tranquilizers, antihistamines, antidepressants, sedatives, sleep inducers, alcohol and narcotics.

Cyclocort® (*Lederle*)
See: Adrenocorticoid Class-Topical

Cyclospasmol® (*Wyeth*)
See: Cyclandelate

Cyproheptadine
See: Antihistamine Class

Cytomel® (*Smith Kline & French*)
See: Thyroid Hormone Class

Dalmane® (*Roche*)
See: Benzodiazepine Class

Danthron
See: Laxative-Stimulant Class

Darvocet-N® (*Lilly*)
See: Acetaminophen
See: Propoxyphene

Darvon® (*Lilly*)
See: Propoxyphene

Darvon Compound® (*Lilly*)
See: APC
See: Acetaminophen
See: Propoxyphene

Decadron® (*Merck Sharp & Dohme*)

See: Adrenocorticoid Class - Systemic

Decadron® Ophthalmic (*Merck Sharp & Dohme*)
See: Adrenocorticoid Class-Systemic and Topical

Decadron®Turbinaire® (*Merck Sharp & Dohme*)
See: Adrenocorticoid Class-Systemic and Topical

Deconamine®-SR(*Berlex*)
See: Pseudoephedrine
See: Antihistamine Class

Deltasone® (*Upjohn*)
See: Adrenocorticoid Class- Systemic

Demerol® Oral (*Winthrop*)
See: Meperidine

Demi-Regroton® (*USV*)
See: Reserpine
See: Rauwolfia Alkaloid Class
See: Thiazide Diuretics

Demulen® (*Searle & Co.*)
See: Estrogen + Progestin   Class

Depakene® (*Abbott*)
See: Valproic Acid

Deserpidine
See: Rauwolfia Alkaloid Class

Desipramine
See: Tricyclic Antidepressant Class

Desonide
See: Adrenocorticoid Class-Topical

Desoximetasone
See: Adrenocorticoid Class-Topical

Desquam-X® Wash (*Westwood*)

Category Of Drug: Anti-bacterial

Ingredients: Benzoyl Peroxide + Sodium Octoxynol-3 Sulfonate + EDTA + Dioctyl Sodium Sulfosuccinate + Magnesium Aluminum Silicate + Methylcellulose

Intended Effects: To treat acne.

Side Effects: Excessive drying, peeling, puffiness, stinging or reddening of the skin.

Warnings: Avoid contact with eyes and mouth. For external use only. Patients known to be sensitive to benzoic acid products and cinnamon may also be sensitive to this drug.

Desyrel® (*Mead Johnson*)
  See: Trazodone

Dexamethasone
  See: Adrenocorticoid Class - Systemic or Topical

Dexchlorpheniramine
  See: Antihistamine Class

Dexedrine®
  See: Amphetamine Class

Dextroamphetamine®
  See: Amphetamine Class

Dextromethorphan

Category Of Drug: Anticough

Intended Effects: To reduce the severity, amount and

duration of coughing from allergic disorders or infections of the bronchial tubes.

Side Effects: Mild drowsiness in sensitive individuals. Skin rash, itching. Rare: indigestion, nausea, dizziness.

Warnings: If drowsiness occurs, drive and operate machinery with great caution. Should be used with caution by people who have bronchial asthma (this drug may aggravate that condition) or people with impaired liver function.

Possible Interactions: If this drug is taken with MAO inhibitor antidepressants, serious side effects may result.

Note: No Rx prescription required

DiaBeta® (*Hoechst-Roussel*)
  See: Antidiabetic

Diabinese® (*Pfizer*)
  See: Antidiabetic Class

Diamox® (*Lederle*)
  See: Acetazolamide

Diazepam
  See: Benzodiazepine Class

Dicloxacillin

See: Penicillin Class

Dicyclomine

Brand Name: Bentyl®

Category Of Drug: Antispasm

Intended Effects: To relieve smooth muscle spasm in the gastrointestinal tract (esophagus, stomach, intestine, colon); to treat infant colic.

Side Effects: Dry mouth, difficulty in urination, blurred vision, heart palpitations, loss of taste, headache, nervousness, drowsiness, weakness, dizziness, sleeplessness, nausea, vomiting, impotence, constipation, bloated feeling, itching, decreased sweating, confusion or excitement.

Warnings: Should not be used by those having bladder or intestinal obstructions, severe ulcers or colitis, or a muscular condition known as myasthenia gravis. Should be used with caution by patients with liver or kidney disease, over-active thyroid, coronary heart disease, high blood pressure, hiatal hernia, or glaucoma. Heat stroke is possible if person is in hot environment. Caution should be used in driving or operating machinery. Nursing mothers may experience difficulty in adequate milk production.

Possible Interactions: The effects of this drug may be increased if taken with antidepressants or antihistamines.

Didrex™ (*Upjohn*)
See: Appetite Suppressant Class

Dienestrol Vaginal Cream.
  See: Estrogen   Class-Vaginal

Diethylpropion
  See: Appetite Suppressant Class

Diethylstilbestrol
  See: Estrogen Class-Systemic

Diflunisal

Brand Name: Dolobid®

Category Of Drug: Pain Reliever, Anti-inflammatory

Intended Effects: To relieve mild to moderate pain, to provide relief from osteoarthritis.

Side Effects: Peptic ulcers, stomach bleeding, nausea, vomiting, indigestion, diarrhea, constipation, gas, inability to sleep, sleepwalking, dizziness, ringing in the ears, skin rash, loss of balance, water retention, headache, tiredness, itching, sweating, dry mucous membranes, weight loss, belching, flushing of the skin, inflammation of the mucous lining of the mouth, nervousness, difficult breathing, awareness of heartbeat, fainting, reduced production of blood cells, visual disturbances, muscle cramps, depression, tingling sensations, difficult or painful urination, chest pain, fever, "unwell" feeling, kidney or liver damage from long use or large doses, allergic symptoms.

Warnings: Use with caution in people with ulcers, bleeding problems, impaired kidney function, poor heart function, high blood pressure, or high water retention. May cause birth defects — use caution during first two trimesters; avoid use during last trimester of pregnancy. Present in mothers' milk — avoid drug or avoid nursing. Should not be used by people taking aspirin or other nonsteroidal anti-inflammatory drugs. Alert doctor to any eye problems. Take with milk, water or meals to reduce stomach upset. Swallow tablets whole — do not crush or chew.

Possible Interactions: Dolobid® increases the level of acetaminophen in the blood — use aspirin only on doctor's advice. Increases the effects of warfarin, acenocoumarol, phenprocoumon, and other oral anticlotting drugs — dosage may need to be adjusted. Indomethacin should be avoided or used with extreme caution to avoid severe stomach bleeding. Decreases the effect of sulindac. May increase the tendency of hydrocholorothiazde and furosemide to increase the uric acid levels in the blood. Increases the elimination rate of naproxen. Antacids reduce the effects of Dolobid®.

Note: See Salicylate Class

Digitalis Class

Generic/Brand Name: Digoxin/Lanoxin®

Category Of Drug: Heart Rhythm Regulator

Intended Effects: To slow and strengthen heartbeat, to correct heart rhythm, to treat congestive heart disease, and to reduce fluid retention.

Side Effects: Loss of appetite, nausea, vomiting, diarrhea, blurred vision, problems with color perception, headache, weakness, apathy, disturbances of heart rhythm, slow pulse.

Warnings: Do not use if heart rate is less than 50 beats per minute — contact doctor immediately. Kidney problems may require reduced dosage. May cause disturbances of heart rhythm in patients with rheumatic heart disease. The use of digitalis to treat obesity may be dangerous since it can cause serious adverse effects which may lead to death. Any illness which causes diarrhea, vomiting, dehydration of liver problems should be reported to physician since this may alter the drug's effectiveness. Known to be present in mothers' milk — avoid drug or avoid nursing.

Possible Interactions: Antibiotics, steroid and thyroid hormones, diuretics, reserpine, ephedrine, or epinephrine may interact with digitalis medicines and cause disturbances in heart rhythm or possible poisoning. Antibiotics may increase rates of absorption and necessitate a decrease in dosage. Dilantin® may alter the body's requirements for digitalis medicines by decreasing the body's requirements at first, and increasing the body's requirements later. Antacids, laxatives, phenobarbital, or phenylbutazone may cause reduced absorption or increased elimination, resulting in a need for higher dosage; consult physician. Any medications affecting the heart may interact with digitalis and require close monitoring by a physician.

Digoxin
See: Digitalis Class

Dilantin® (*Parke-Davis*)
See: Phenytoin

Dilantin® + Phenobarbital (*Parke-Davis*)
See: Barbiturate Class
See: Phenytoin

Dimetane® Expectorant (*Robins*)

Category Of Drug: Anticough, Phlegm Loosener, Antihistamine

Ingredients: Brompheniramine + Guaifenesin + Phenylephrine + Phenylpropanolamine + Alcohol.

Intended Effects: To relieve coughing and loosen phlegm.

Side Effects: Skin rash, itching, drowsiness, indigestion, nausea, headache, low or high blood pressure, sedation, sleepiness, fatigue, confusion, nervousness, dry mouth, nose or throat.

Warnings: Antihistamines should not be used to treat lower respiratory tract symptoms including asthma. Known to be present in mothers' milk — avoid drug or avoid nursing. May cause birth defects in humans — avoid during first three months of pregnancy. May cause excitability in children. Should be used with caution by people with peptic ulcer, narrow angle glaucoma, prostate or bladder problems, high blood pressure, heart disease. Use caution while driving if this drug causes drowsiness.

Possible Interactions: MAO inhibitor antidepressants intensify and prolong the drying effects of antihistamines. Sedation may increase when taken with: tranquilizers, antidepressants, sedatives, sleep inducers, alcohol and narcotics.

Dimetane® Expectorant-DC (*Robins*)
See: Codeine
See: Dimetane Expectorant

Dimetane Extentabs® (*Robins*)
See: Antihistamine Class

Dimetapp® (*Robins*)

Category Of Drug: Antihistamine, Decongestant

Ingredients: Brompheniramine + Phenylephrine + Phenylpropanolamine

Intended Effects: To relieve sinus, nose and throat congestion caused by hay fever, sinusitis, and infections.

Side Effects: Allergic rash in sensitive individuals, dryness of nose, throat and mouth, drowsiness, nervousness, insomnia, tiredness, giddiness, chest tightness, headache, faintness, dizziness, visual disturbances, incoordination, increase in blood pressure.

Warnings: Use with caution in people with heart disease or high blood pressure. Causes birth defects in animals —

avoid during first three months of pregnancy. Known to be present in mothers' milk — avoid drug or avoid nursing. Tablets not for children under 12. People using this drug should drive and operate machinery with caution. People allergic to other antihistamines may also be allergic to this drug. Do not exceed recommended dose — large doses can lead to serious rise in blood pressure.

Possible Interactions: If given with MAO inhibitor antidepressants, serious rise in blood pressure may occur. Sedation may increase when taken with: tranquilizers, antihistamines, antidepressants, sedatives, sleep inducers, alcohol and narcotics.

Note: No Rx prescription required

Diphenhydramine
See: Antihistamine Class

Dipivefrin

Brand Name: Propine®

Category Of Drug: Antiglaucoma

Intended Effects: To control pressure within the eye in chronic open-angle glaucoma.

Side Effects: Frequent (6%): burning, stinging or other eye irritation. Rare: unusually fast or irregular heartbeat, high blood pressure.

Warnings: Do not exceed recommended dosage.

Physician may recommend regular eye pressure exams during therapy with this drug.

Diprosone® (*Schering*)
See: Adrenocorticoid   Class-Topical

Dipyridamole

Brand Name: Persantine®

Category Of Drug: Blood Vessel Enlarger

Intended Effects: To dilate or enlarge coronary arteries and increase blood flow to the heart. To prevent the pain of angina pectoris, but not to stop an acute anginal attack. To improve exercise tolerance.

Side Effects: Headache, dizziness, nausea, flushing or reddening of the skin, weakness, blackouts, upset stomach, skin rash and possible aggravation of angina at the start of therapy.

Disalcid® (*Riker*)
See: Salsalate
See: Salicylate Class

Disopyramide Phosphate

Brand Name: Norpace®

Category Of Drug: Heart Rhythm Regulator

Intended Effects: To regulate heart action, to reduce disturbances of heart rhythm.

Side Effects: In clinical trials, the following reactions have been reported in the percentages given: dry mouth (32%), difficult urination (14%), constipation (11%). Frequent (3-9%): blurred vision, dry nose, eyes or throat, frequent urination, stomach or intestinal pain, bloating or gas, dizziness, fatigue, muscle weakness, headache, uneasiness, aches and pains. Less frequent (1-3%): urinary retention, impotence, low blood pressure, congestive heart failure, fluid retention, weight gain, shortness of breath, blackouts, chest pain, loss of appetite, diarrhea, vomiting, rashes, itching, nervousness, high blood levels of potassium, cholesterol and triglycerides. Infrequent (less than 1%): depression, insomnia, difficult urination, tingling sensations, metabolic disorders. Rare: acute psychosis.

Warnings: Effectiveness of this drug should be closely monitored by a physician. May stimulate contractions of the pregnant uterus. Should be used with extreme caution by patients with glaucoma, myasthenia gravis, urinary retention. Reduce dosage in people with poor kidney or liver function. Known to be present in mothers' milk — avoid drug or avoid nursing.

Possible Interactions: May interact with other drugs which affect heart rhythm such as lidocaine, propranolol, procainamide, and quinidine. Alcohol may increase the blood-pressure lowering effect of this drug.

Disulfiram

Category Of Drug: Anti-alcoholism

Intended Effects: To aid in the treatment of alcoholism by making patients nauseous after drinking alcohol.

Side Effects: The following side effects are **intended** to make people avoid alcohol. They should **only occur** when patients consume alcohol. Flushing, throbbing in the head and neck, throbbing headache, nausea, severe vomiting, sweating, thirst, chest pain, respiratory difficulty, weakness, blurred vision, confusion. Occasional skin rashes, impaired vision, pain, weakness, tingling in the limbs.

Warnings: Should never be given to a patient who has consumed alcohol within the past 12 hours. Patient (and relatives) should be informed of side effects before medication is taken. Alcohol in any form including sauces, cough mixtures, aftershave lotions, backrubs or alcoholic beverages, even in small amounts, must be completely avoided during and for 14 days after therapy with Antabuse® to avoid alcohol-antabuse reaction. Not for patients who have heart disease, for those taking metronidazole (Flagyl®). Should be used with extreme caution by people with diabetes, epilepsy, underactive thyroid, brain damage, kidney infection, cirrhosis of the liver.

Possible Interactions: Over-the-counter cough syrups, may cause alcohol-antabuse reaction. Should be used with caution in patients receiving phenytoin — adjustment of phenytoin dosage may be necessary. May increase the effects of anticlotting drugs, barbiturates, diazepam. If taken with isoniazid or metronidazole (Flagyl®) behavioral and mental disturbances may occur.

Ditropan® (*Marion*)
See: Oxybutynin

Diulo™ (*Searle*)
See: Thiazide Diuretic Class

Diupres® (*Merck Sharp & Dohme*)
See: Rauwolfia   Alkaloid Class
See: Thiazide Diuretic Class

Diuril® (*Merck Sharp & Dohme*)
See: Thiazide Diuretic Class

Dolobid® (*Merck Sharp & Dohme*)
See: Diflunisal

Donnagel®-PG (*Robins*)

Category Of Drug: Antidiarrhea, Narcotic

Ingredients: Kaolin + Pectin + Hyoscyamine + Atropine + Hyoscine + Opium

Intended Effects: To treat diarrhea, intestinal cramping; to relieve acute stomach upsets, gastritis and nausea.

Side Effects: Blurred vision, dry mouth, flushing, dry skin, difficult urination, mild drowsiness.

Warnings: Should be used with care by people with glaucoma or urinary bladder neck obstruction. Should not be used by people with advanced liver or kidney disease. Because this drug contains opium, it may be habit forming in large doses. Known to be present in mothers' milk — avoid drug or avoid nursing. Causes birth defects in animals — avoid during first three months of pregnancy.

Possible Interactions: Sedation may increase when taken with: tranquilizers, antihistamines, antidepressants, sedatives, sleep inducers, alcohol and narcotics.

Donnatal® (*Robins*)

Category Of Drug: Antispasm, Sedative, Nervous-System Regulator

Ingredients: Phenobarbital + Hyoscyamine Sulfate + Atropine Sulfate + Hyoscine Hydrobromide

Intended Effects: To treat spasms associated with irritable bowels and acute enterocolitis.

Side Effects: Dry mouth, urinary problems, blurred vision, rapid or pounding heartbeat, dilated pupils, increased pressure within the eyeball, loss of taste, headache, nervousness, drowsiness, weakness, agitation, dizziness, insomnia, nausea, vomiting, impotence, interruption in milk flow in nursing mothers, constipation, bloating, muscle and bone aches, shock, hives, skin rashes, decreased sweating, excitement.

Warnings: Sudden withdrawal can cause feelings of anxiety, delirium or convulsions. Decreased sweating may lead to heat prostration. Treatment should not be used in cases of possible intestinal obstruction, especially in those who have had recent intestinal surgery. Prolonged use of phenobarbital may be habit-forming or addictive; should not be given to peoplewho are addiction prone. Should not be used in cases of glaucoma, bladder neck obstruction, poor heart function, ulcerative colitis, myasthenia gravis, hiatal hernia, porphyria. Known to be present in mothers' milk — avoid drug or avoid nursing.

Possible Interactions: May increase the action of anti-clotting drugs and cause bleeding. Sedation may increase when taken with: tranquilizers, antihistamines, antidepressants, sedatives, sleep inducers, alcohol and narcotics. Phenylbutazone, laxatives and antacids may decrease the effects of this drug. Propranolol and quinidine may increase the effects of this drug.

Donnazyme® (*Robins*)

Category Of Drug: Nervous-System Regulator, Anti-spasm

Ingredients: Pancreatin + Pepsin + Bile Salts + hyoscyamine Sulfate + Atropine Sulfate + Hyoscine Hydrobromide + Phenobarbital

Intended Effects: To relieve symptoms associated with "nervous indigestion" and other gastrointestinal disorders, to treat decreased digestive enzyme secretion.

Side Effects: Difficult urination, decreased sweating, excitement, blurred vision, increased eyeball pressure, loss of taste, headache, nervousness, drowsiness, weakness, dizziness, nausea, vomiting, impotence, constipation, joint pain, decreased ability to produce milk. In the elderly, even small doses may result in excitement, agitation, or drowsiness.

Warnings: Do not drive or operate machinery if drowsiness occurs. Use with caution by people with kidney or liver disease, over-active thyroid, heart disease, congestive heart failure, irregular heartbeat, high blood pressure. Should not be given to people with a history of dependence upon drugs. Should not be discontinued abruptly in case of addiction to avoid convulsions. In hot weather, heat prostration may occur because of decreased sweating. Not for people with glaucoma, bladder neck obstruction, severe ulcerative colitis, myasthenia gravis, hiatal hernia, iliostomy or colostomy. Known to be present in mothers' milk — avoid drug or avoid nursing.

Possible Interactions: May decrease effects of anticlotting drugs. Sedation may increase when taken with: tranquilizers, antihistamines, antidepressants, sedatives, sleep inducers, alcohol and narcotics.

Doriden® (*USV*)
 See: Glutethimide

Doxepin
 See: Tricyclic Antidepressant Class

Doxidan® (*Hoechst-Roussel*)
 See: Laxatives-Emollient Class
 See: Laxatives-Stimulant Class

Doxycycline
See: Tetracycline Class

Drixoral® (*Schering*)

Category Of Drug: Antihistamine, Decongestant

Ingredients: Dexbrompheniramine + Pseudoephedrine Sulfate

Intended Effects: To relieve nasal and bronchial congestion in cases of allergy, runny nose, and blockage of the eustachian tube.

Side Effects: Drowsiness is the most frequent side effect. Less frequent: hives, rashes, shock, sensitivity to light, excessive perspiration, chills, dryness of the mouth, nose, and throat, disturbances in heartbeat, low blood pressure, anemia and other blood disorders, sedation, dizziness, loss of balance, ringing in the ears, disturbed coordination, fatigue, confusion, restlessness, excitation, nervousness, tremor, irritability, insomnia, elevated mood, tingling sensations, blurred vision, hysteria, generalized pain symptoms, convulsions, upset stomach, loss of appetite, nausea, vomiting, diarrhea, constipation, urinary problems, early menstruation, thickening of bronchial secretions, tightness of chest, wheezing, nasal stuffiness, fear, headache, weakness, difficulty in breathing, angina pectoris, high blood pressure, hallucinations.

Warnings: Do not use in cases of sensitivity to other bronchial tube relaxers or antihistamines. Should not be used with MAO inhibitor antidepressants. Should not be used in

120

cases of high blood pressure, severe heart disease or over-active thyroid. Should be used cautiously in cases of glaucoma, peptic ulcer, stomach or duodenal blockage. Should not be used during pregnancy, because use in the third trimester of pregnancy may cause severe reactions such as convulsions in newborn and premature infants. Small amounts of the drug may be passed in milk from mothers to infants. Avoid drug or avoid nursing. Many other over-the-counter medicines for colds react unfavorably with this drug.

Possible Interactions: Sedation may increase when taken with: tranquilizers, antihistamines, antidepressants, sedatives, sleep inducers, alcohol and narcotics. May inhibit the action of oral anticoagulants. May react with MAO inhibitors to produce extremely high blood pressure, possibly leading to death. Pseudoephedrine should not be used with ganglionic blocking drugs such as mecamylamine hydrochloride or with beta- adrenergic blocking agents, since it reduces the blood pressure-lowering effect of these drugs. May interfere with heart rhythm when used with digitalis. May enter the blood stream rapidly when taken with antacids.

Note: No Rx prescription required

Dulcolax® (*Boehringer*)
  See: Laxatives -Stimulant Class

Duofilm® (*Stiefel*)

Category Of Drug: Caustic
Ingredients: Salicylic Acid + Lactic Acid + Flexible

Collodion

Intended Effects: To treat and remove common warts.

Side Effects: Irritation of skin surrounding warts if drug touches this area.

Warnings: Should not be used by diabetics or by people with impaired blood circulation. Not for use on birthmarks, moles or unusual warts with hair growing from them. Do not permit Duofilm® to contact mucous membranes, eyes, or normal skin surrounding warts. Discontinue treatment if extreme irritation occurs. This drug is highly flammable.

Possible Interactions: Do not use with acne medications applied to the skin.

Note: Over-the-counter drugs with similar formulas are available.

Duricef® (*Mead Johnson*)
  See: Cephalosporin Class

DV® Cream (*Merrell Dow*)
  See: Estrogen-Vaginal

Dyazide® (*Smith Kline & French*)
  See: Thiazide Diuretic Class
  See: Triamterene

Dymelor® (*Lily*)
See: Antidiabetic Class

Dyphylline
See: Xanthine Class

Dyrenium® (*Smith Kline & French*)
See: Triamterene

E.E.S.® (*Abbott*)
See: Erythromycin Class

Effersyllium® (*Stuart*)
See: Laxatives-Bulk Class

Note: No Rx prescription required

Elavil® (*Merck Sharp & Dohme*)
See: Tricyclic Antidepressant Class

Elixophyllin® (*Berlex*)
See: Xanthine Class

Empirin® + Codeine (*Burroughs Wellcome*)
See: Salicylate Class

See: Codeine

E-Mycin® (*Upjohn*)
See: Erythromycin Class

Enalapril
See: Angiotensin Converting Enzyme Inhibitor Class

Enduron® (*Abbott*)
See: Thiazide Diuretic Class

Enduronyl® (*Abbott*)
See: Thiazide Diuretic Class
See: Rauwolfia Alkaloid Class

Enovid® (*Searle*)
See: Estrogen + Progestin Class

Entex® (*Norwich Eaton*)

Category Of Drug: Decongestant

Ingredients: Phenylpropanolamine Hydrochloride + Guaifenesin

Intended Effects: To relieve swollen mucous membranes of the entire respiratory tract, to improve sinus and eustachian tube drainage.

Side Effects: Nervousness, insomnia, restlessness, headache, stomach irritation. Possible urinary retention in patients with enlarged prostate.

Warnings: Should be used with caution by people with high blood pressure, glaucoma, diabetes, heart disease, overactive thyroid, vascular disease. Not for children under the age of 12.

Possible Interactions: May cause serious rise in blood pressure if taken with MAO inhibitors. Many over-the-counter drugs for coughs, allergies and colds may react unfavorably with this drug.

Epsom Salts
See: Laxatives-HyperosmoticClass

Equagesic® *(Wyeth)*

Category Of Drug: Tranquilizer, Pain Reliever

Ingredients: Meprobamate + Ethoheptazine Citrate + Aspirin

Intended Effects: To relieve pain in muscle and bone diseases or tension headache.

Side Effects: Drowsiness, dizziness, nausea, vomiting, loss of balance, skin rash, fever, fainting spells, bronchial spasms, blood disorders, incoordinated movements.

Warnings: Causes birth defects in animals — avoid during first three months of pregnancy. Known to be present in mothers' milk — avoid drug or avoid nursing. Not for children under 12. Drug dependence may develop with high doses over long period of time. Drive with caution since this drug may impair mental alertness. Use alcohol with extreme caution. After extended use, discontinue gradually with physician's guidance to avoid convulsions. Not for people with previous sensitivity to aspirin, meprobamate or ethoheptazine citrate.

Possible Interactions: May decrease the effects of oral anticlotting drugs. Seizure patterns may be changed if this drug is taken with anticonvulsants. Sedation may increase when taken with tranquilizers, antihistamines, antidepressants, sedatives, sleep inducers, alcohol and narcotics.

Equanil® *(Wyeth)*
See: Meprobamate

Ergot Mesylates

Brand Name: Hydergine®

Category Of Drug: Antisenility

Intended Effects: To increase circulation to the brain and to increase its rate of oxygen use; to combat symptoms of senility like confusion, mood-depression, unsociability, reduced alertness, poor memory. Unlike natural ergot alkaloids (which are used to treat migraine headaches), it does not constrict arteries leading to the brain.

Side Effects: Upset stomach, mouth irritation, and digestive disturbances. Rare (usually occurring only with

overdoses): low blood pressure, slow heartbeat and headache.

Warnings: People who have a known sensitivity to this
drug should avoid its use. Should be used with caution by
people with low pulse rates.

Possible Interactions: May interact with blood- pressure reducers, or heart rhythm regulators to cause a drop in
blood pressure or excessively slow heart rate.

ERYC® (*Parke-Davis*)
  See: Erythromycin Class

Erythrocin® (*Abbott*)
  See: Erythromycin Class

Erythromycin Class

Generic / Brand Names:
  Erythromycin/ E-Mycin®, ERYC®, Pediamycin®
  Erythromycin estolate/Ilosone®
  Erythromycin ethylsuccinate/E.E.S.®
  Erythromycin stearate/Erythrocin®

Category Of Drug: Antibiotic

Intended Effects: To combat infections caused by certain
bacteria.

Side Effects: Stomach cramps and discomfort, nausea,

vomiting, diarrhea, skin rash, liver damage. Fungus or other infections may develop with prolonged use. Rare: shock.

Warnings: Should be used with caution by patients with kidney or liver disease. Not for people who have had allergic reactions to any form of this drug. E-Mycin® tablets are enteric-coated to dissolve in the bowels rather than the stomach and reduce stomach discomfort.

Possible Interactions: Increases the effect of theophylline and methyl-prednisolone — dosage may need to be adjusted.

Esidrix® (*CIBA*)
  See: Thiazide Diuretic Class

Eskalith® (*Smith Kline & French*)
  See: Lithium

Estrogen Class-Systemic

Generic / Brand Names:
  Conjugated Estrogen/Premarin®
  Diethylstilbestrol/Stilphostrol®
  Estropipate/Ogen®

Category Of Drug: Female Hormones

Intended Effects: To treat the symptoms of menopause, to supplement the body's production of estrogens in cases of estrogen deficiency during the menopause and after the removal of ovaries, to treat certain cancers in women and men, to treat infertility, to prevent painful swelling of the breasts after pregnancy in women who choose not to nurse their babies.

Side Effects: Most common: nausea. Less frequent: vomiting, breast enlargement and tenderness, benign tumors of the uterus, tumors of the liver, jaundice, fluid retention, abnormal bleeding from the vagina, headache, dizziness, faintness, changes in vision, breast lumps, mental depression, muscle cramps.

Warnings: May increase the chances of cancer of the endometrium uterus, breasts, cervix, vagina or liver. Should not be taken if cancer is present, except for treatment of certain cancers that spread. May increase the chances of gallbladder disease and abnormal blood clotting. If taken during pregnancy may increase the chance of birth defects or the chance of the development of cancer of the vagina or cervix later in the life of the child. Should be used with caution by people with asthma, epilepsy, mental depression, migraine headaches, cystic disease of the breast, history of endometriosis, porphyria, high blood pressure, history of cancer of the breast or reproductive organs, fibroid tumors of the uterus, diabetes, gallbladder disease, kidney disease.

Possible Interactions: Sedatives, tranquilizers and phenytoin may decrease the effectiveness of estrogens.

Estrogen Class-Vaginal

Generic/Brand Names:
  Conjugated Estrogen/Premarin® Vaginal Cream
  Dienestrol/DV® Cream
  Estropipate/Ogen® Vaginal Cream

Category Of Drug: Female Hormone

Intended Effects: To treat the shrinking and irritation of the vagina or vulva following menopause or removal of ovaries.

Side Effects: See Estrogen-Systemic

Warnings: See Estrogen-Systemic. Use at bedtime to increase absorption. May be absorbed through the penis during intercourse and cause tenderness and enlargement of male breast tissue.

Possible Interactions: See Estrogen-Systemic

Estrogen + Progestin Class

Generic / Brand Names:
Ethynodiol Diacetate + Ethinyl Estradiol/Demulen®
Ethynodiol Diacetate + Mestranol/Ovulen®
Levonorgestrel + Ethinyl Estradiol/Triphasil 21®
Norethindrone + Ethinyl Estradiol/Brevicon®, Loestrin®, Loestrin®FE,Modicon®,Norinyl®(1+35),Norlestrin®, Nor- lestrin®FE, Ortho- Novum® (1/35 or 10/11), Ovcon®.
Norethindrone + Mestranol/Ortho-Novum® (1/50 or 1/80 or 2), Norinyl® (1+50 or 1+80 or 2)
Norethynodrel + Mestranol/Enovid®
Norgestrel + Ethinyl Estradiol/ Lo/Ovral®, Ovral®

Intended Effects: To prevent ovulation and pregnancy, to supplement the body's production of hormones. Effectiveness is higher than with other means of contraception. Certain brand names contain smaller amounts of hormones than other brand names, consequently they are slightly less effective, but their side effects are reduced. These low dosage combinations are still more effective than other methods of birth control.

Side Effects: Decrease in milk production, tenderness of the breasts, irregular menstruation, spotting, irritability, high blood pressure, headache, depression, masculinization, growth of facial hair, skin rashes, increased sensitivity to contact lenses, visual disturbances with halos around lights, pains in the joints and muscles, fluid retention, and general discomfort.

Warnings: Worsening of migraine, epilepsy, asthma, kidney or heart disease is possible because of increased water retention. Not for those with history of phlebitis, stroke, angina, heart attack, blood clots, impaired liver function or liver disease, history of cancer of the reproductive organs or the breast, unexplained and abnormal vaginal bleeding. Should be used with caution by patients with cystic breast disease, endometriosis, high blood pressure, asthma, epilepsy, diabetes, migraine headaches, fibroid tumors of the uterus, mental depression, gallbladder disease or gallstones. Known to be present in mothers' milk — avoid drug or avoid nursing. Causes birth defects — avoid during pregnancy. Extended use of oral contraceptives may lead to gradual rise in blood pressure, gall bladder disease, increased growth of fibroid tumors of the uterus, delayed return to normal menstruation, increased rates of ectopic or tubal pregnancies, and delayed pregnancy after oral contraceptives are discontinued, especially in women with irregular menstrual cycles. Women who use oral contraceptives should not smoke; cigarette smoking by oral contraceptive users increases the risk of serious side effects of the heart and blood vessels. This risk increases with age (especially over 35) and with heavy smoking.

Possible Interactions: Ampicillin, some antihistamines, meprobamate, phenobarbital, phenytoin, rifampin, tetracycline, chloramphenicol, or high blood-pressure medicines may decrease the effects of oral contraceptives. Oral contraceptives may decrease the effects of oral anticlotting drugs.

Estropipate
See: Estrogen Class-Systemic

Ethynodiol Diacetate + Ethinyl Estradiol
See: Estrogen + Progestin Class

Ethynodiol Diacetate + Mestranol
See: Estrogen + Progestin Class

Etrafon® (*Schering*)
See: Phenothiazine Class
See: Tricyclic Antidepressant Class

Euthroid® (*Parke-Davis*)
See: Thyroid Hormone Class

Eutonyl® (*Abbott*)
See: Monoamine Oxidase (MAO) Inhibitor Class

Eutron® (*Abbott*)
See: Monoamine Oxidase (MAO) Inhibitor Class

Ex-Lax® (*Ex-Lax Pharmaceutical*)
See: Laxatives-Stimulant Class

Note: No Rx prescription required

Fastin® (*Beecham*)
See: Appetite Suppressant Class

Note: No Rx prescription required

Feldene® (*Pfizer*)
See: Piroxicam

Fenoprofen

Brand Name: Nalfon®

Category Of Drug: Anti-inflammatory, Pain Reliever, Fever Reducer

Intended Effects: To relieve inflammation, pain and fever of rheumatoid arthritis and osteoarthritis, to relieve mild to moderate pain.

Side Effects: Most frequent (3-9%): constipation, nausea, vomiting, dizziness, itching, throbbing heartbeat, nervousness, weakness. Less frequent (1-3%): abdominal pain, loss of appetite, blood in the stool, diarrhea, gas, dry mouth, tremor, confusion, insomnia, rash, increased sweating, hives, ringing in the ears, blurred vision, decreased hearing, rapid heartbeat, shortness of breath, fatigue, feelings of uneasiness. Infrequent (less than 1%): upset stomach, peptic ulcer, jaundice, hepatitis, difficult urination and inflammation within the urinary tract, bleeding under the skin, bruising, blood disorders. Unconfirmed but reported: hive-like allergic reaction within the mouth, loss of hair, inflammation of pancreas, ulcers in the mouth, disturbances in heart rhythm, depression, disorientation, seizures, inflammation of cranial nerves, burning tongue, double vision, pain behind the eye, anemia, personality change, inflammation of the lymph nodes and mastoid bone fever.

Warnings: Not for people who are sensitive to other anti-inflammatory drugs such as aspirin. Not for people with poor kidney function. Should be used with great caution by people with active peptic ulcer, stomach or intestinal bleeding, high blood pressure, or poor heart function. Consult physician if jaundice occurs. Not for children under the age of 14. Use caution while driving or operating machinery if drowsiness occurs.

Possible Interactions: Aspirin, aspirin-containing medicines and phenobarbital may decrease its effects. May increase effects of hydantoin, sulfonamides, sulfonylureas and anticlotting drugs, causing bleeding.

Feosol® (*Smith Kline & French*)
See: Ferrous Sulfate

Note: No Rx prescription required

Fero-Folic-500 (*Abbott*)

Category Of Drug: Vitamin/Mineral Supplement

Ingredients: Ferrous Sulfate + Ascorbic Acid + Niacin + Calcium + Thiamine + Riboflavin + Vitamin B6 + Folic Acid + Vitamin B12 +

Intended Effects: To treat iron deficiency and prevent accompanying folic acid deficiency in nonpregnant adults. In pregnancy: to prevent and treat iron deficiency and to maintain a supply of folic acid.

Side Effects: May cause gray or black discoloration of stools (normal). Stomach upset, (which may be reduced by taking this drug following a meal). Increased allergic reactions have been reported.

Warnings: Not for people with pernicious anemia, and those rare people who are sensitive to folic acid. Not for use by children. Folic acid, ascorbic acid and B-complex vitamins are present in breast — nursing mothers should take only under physician's recommendation.

Possible Interactions: May decrease the effects of tetracyclines. The antiparkinsonism effects of levodopa may be reversed. Eggs, milk, and whole grain cereals inhibit the absorption of iron. Magnesium trisilicate and antacids containing carbonates decrease the absorption of iron.

Ferro-Sequels® (*Lederle*)

See: Ferrous Sulfate

Note: No Rx prescription required

Ferrous Sulfate (Iron)

Brand Names: Feosol®, Ferro-Sequels®

Category Of Drug: Mineral Supplement

Intended Effects: To prevent or correct iron-deficiency anemia. To supplement iron lost in blood at menstruation.

Side Effects: Stomach pain, soreness or cramps, diarrhea, nausea, vomiting, constipation, heartburn. Stomach upset may be reduced if this drug is taken with food. If taken by mouth, darkening of stools or teeth may result (normal).

Warnings: People with iron-deficiency anemia, should take iron supplements only under physician's guidance. Not for people with hemolytic anemia. Use with caution in people with ulcerative colitis, peptic ulcer, previous stomach surgery, or alcohol addiction. Should not be taken in cases of acute hepatitis or if known iron deposits are present in the body. Excessive amounts of iron can be toxic to the body. Iron supplements should be discontinued once body levels are restored to normal.

Possible Interactions: Eggs, milk, whole grain cereals, magnesium trisilicate and antacids containing carbonate impair the absorption of iron. Iron interferes with the absorption of tetracyclines and vitamin C. Iron preparations taken with allopurinol may cause build-up of iron in the liver.

Fioricet® (*Sandoz*)

Category Of Drug: Pain Reliever, Muscle Relaxer

Ingredients: Butalbital + Acetaminophen + Caffeine

Intended Effects: To relieve pain of tension headache, caused by muscle contraction/spasms.

Side Effects: Drowsiness, dizziness, lightheadedness, nausea, vomiting, flatulence. An overdose or intolerance can cause mental confusion or depression.

Warnings: May be habit forming. The dosage should not be increased without the doctor's permission. Not for people with porphyria (rare blood disorder). Should be used with great caution by people who are mentally depressed, have suicidal tendencies or a history of drug abuse. May cause excitement, depression or confusion in elderly or debilitated people. May be present in mothers' milk — avoid drug or avoid nursing. Drive and operate machinery with caution.

Possible Interactions: Sedation may increase when taken with: tranquilizers, antihistamines, antidepressants, sedatives, sleep inducers, alcohol and narcotics. Butalbital decreases the effectiveness of anticlotting drugs and antidepressants.

Note: See Acetaminophen
   See Barbiturate Class

Fiorinal® (*Sandoz*)

Category Of Drug: Pain Reliever, Sedative, Muscle Relaxant

Ingredients: Aspirin + Caffeine + Butalbital

Intended Effects: To relieve mild to moderate pain, especially in tension (muscle contraction) headache.

Side Effects: Dizziness, drowsiness, lightheadedness, nausea, vomiting.

Warnings: Not for people with porphyria. Psychological and physical dependence and kidney damage may occur if high doses are taken over a long period of time. Should be used with extreme caution by people with peptic ulcer, blood clotting problems or kidney disease. Not for children under the age of 12. Known to be present in mothers' milk — avoid drug or avoid nursing. Drive or operate machinery with caution.

Possible Interactions: Sedation may increase when taken with: tranquilizers, antihistamines, antidepressants, sedatives, sleep inducers, alcohol and narcotics.

Note: See Barbiturate Class
See Salicylate Class

Fiorinal® + Codeine (*Sandoz*)
See: Fiorinal®
See: Codeine

Flagyl® (*Searle*)
See: Metronidazole

Flexeril® (*Merck Sharp & Dohme*)
  See: Cyclobenzaprine

Fluocinolone
  See: Adrenocorticoid Class-Topical

Fluocinonide
  See: Adrenocorticoid Class-Topical

Fluorometholone
  See: Adrenocorticoid Class-Topical

Fluoride

Brand Name: Luride®

Category Of Drug: Vitamin/Mineral Supplement

Intended Effects: To aid in protecting teeth from cavities.

Side Effects: Rare: allergic rash.

Warnings: Not for children under the age of three. Should not be taken where the fluoride content of drinking water is more than 0.3ppm — check with pharmacist or dentist for fluoride content of water in your area.

Possible Interactions: Fluoride should not be taken with dairy products, since this combination may produce calcium fluoride which is poorly absorbed.

Fluphenazine
See: Phenothiazine Class

Flurandrenolide
See: Adrenocorticoid Class-Topical

Flurazepam
See: Benzodiazepine Class

FML® Liquifilm® (*Allergan*)

Category Of Drug: Anti-infective

Ingredients: Fluorometholone + Polyvinyl Alcohol + Benzalkonium Chloride + Edetate Disodium + Sodium Chloride + Sodium Phosphate + Monohydrate + Sodium Phosphate Dibasic + Anhydrous + Polysorbate 80 + Purified Water + Sodium Hydroxide

Intended Effects: To treat eye inflammation.

Side Effects: Prolonged treatment may cause glaucoma, damage to the optic nerve, defects in vision, cataracts, secondary infections of the eye from fungus or viruses. In eye diseases which cause thinning of the cornea or sclera, damage to the eye may occur.

Warnings: Not for those with active herpes infections or cold sores, fungus or virus diseases of the eye or tuberculosis of the eye. Treatment may mask or activate infection of the eye.

See: Adrenocorticoid Class-Topical

Folic Acid

Category Of Drug: Vitamin Supplement

Intended Effects: To treat certain types of anemias (megaloblastic) due to folic acid deficiency which often occurs druing pregnancy, infancy or childhood or results from poor nutrition.

Side Effects: Large doses may cause yellow coloring of urine which is not considered a medical problem.

Warnings: This drug is not for treatment of other types of anemias. Diagnosis of pernicious anemia should be ruled out before treatment with folic acid begins. Dosage may need to be increased for alcoholics, people with chronic infection, those on anticonvulsant therapy or those with hemolytic anemia.

Possible Interactions: Long-term use of pain relievers, adrenal hormones, oral contraceptives, or anticonvulsants may decrease the effectiveness of this vitamin.

Furosemide

Brand Name: Lasix®

Category Of Drug: Diuretic, Blood-Pressure Reducer

Intended Effects: To reduce fluid retention and the extra load that it places on the body's circulatory system. To reduce high blood pressure.

Side Effects: Loss of appetite, stomach and mouth irritation, nausea, vomiting, cramping, diarrhea, constipation, jaundice, inflammation of the pancreas, dizziness, vertigo, tingling sensations, headache, blurred vision, ringing in the ears, hearing loss, anemia and other blood disorders, bleeding under the skin, rashes (including light-sensitive rashes), itching, inflammation of the blood vessels, low blood pressure, high blood sugar, muscle spasms, weakness, restlessness, blood clots, pain in the bladder.

Warnings: Physician may recommend diet high in potassium. People allergic to sulfonamides may also be allergic to furosemide. Causes birth defects in animals — avoid during pregnancy. Probably present in mothers' milk — avoid drug or avoid nursing. Should be used with caution by people with diabetes, gout, impaired hearing, liver or kidney disease, impaired kidney or liver function, or those taking any form of insulin, digitalis, cortisone, or oral antidiabetic drugs. Use alcohol with extreme caution.

Possible Interactions: Aspirin and acetaminophen may be eliminated at a slower rate, so their concentrations could build up to harmful levels. Reduces the effect of tubocurarine and increases the effect of succinylcholine. Lithium may build up to harmful levels when taking furosemide. Cephaloridine may have increased harmful effects when taking furosemide. May decrease arterial responsiveness to norepinephrine. Furosemide's effectiveness may be reduced by indomethacin. May increase the effects of other blood-pressure reducers.

Gamma Benzene Hexachloride
See: Lindane

Gantanol®(*Roche*)
See: Sulfonamide Class-Systemic

Gantrisin® (*Roche*)
See: Sulfonamide Class-Systemic
See: Sulfonamide Class-Topical

Garamycin® (*Schering*)
See: Gentamicin - Topical

Gaviscon® (*Marion*)

Category Of Drug: Antacid

Ingredients: Aluminum Hydroxide Dried Gel + Magnesium Trisilicate + Sucrose + Alginic Acid + Sodium Bicarbonate + Starch + Calcium Stearate + Flavoring

Intended Effects: To temporarily relieve sour stomach, heartburn and acid indigestion.

Side Effects: Mild constipation, diarrhea, belching.

Warnings: Not for those on sodium-restricted diets. Should be used with caution by those with kidney disease or reduced kidney function, high blood pressure, frequent diarrhea or constipation. Not for those people taking a prescription antibiotic which contains any form of tetracycline. Chew tablets, do not swallow them whole. Take after meals and drink with water to avoid intestinal obstruction. Do not exceed recommended dose.

Possible Interactions: Antacids may decrease the absorption of tetracyclines if they are taken together.

Note: No Rx prescription required

Garamycin® (*Schering*)
See: Gentamicin - Topical

Gentamicin - Topical

Brand Names: Garamycin®-ophthalmic, Garamycin®-dermatologic

Category Of Drug: Antibiotic

Intended Effects: To treat bacterial infections of the external eye.

Side Effects: Occasional burning or stinging.

Warnings: Prolonged use of topical antibiotics may cause fungus infections. Ointments for the eye may hinder corneal healing.

Geocillin® (*Roerig*)
See: Penicillin Class

Glipizide
See: Antidiabetic Class

Glucotrol® (*Roerig*)
See: Antidiabetic Class

Glutethimide

Brand Name: Doriden®

Category Of Drug: Sleeping Aid, Sedative

Intended Effects: To help control insomnia.

Side Effects: Nausea, blurring of vision, excitation, skin rash, headache, mental confusion, vomiting, slurred speech, dizziness.

Warnings: Impairs mental alertness or physical coordination — do not drive or operate machinery while taking this drug. For short-term use only, since dependence may occur. Known to be present in mothers' milk — avoid drug or avoid nursing.

Possible Interactions: Dosages of some anticlotting-drugs may need to be adjusted if taken with this drug. Sedation may increase when taken with; tranquilizers, antihistamines, antidepressants, sedatives, sleep inducers, alcohol and narcotics.

Glyburide

See: Antidiabetic Class

Granulex (*Hickam*)

Category Of Drug: Skin healing aid

Ingredients: Trypsin + Balsam Peru + Castor Oil + Emulsifier.

Intended Effects: To treat certain skin ulcers, burns, sunburn, wounds; to remove dead or unhealthy tissue and to promote healing.

Warnings: Do not spray on fresh arterial clots or in eyes. Keep out of reach of children. Deliberately concentrating and inhaling the contents can be harmful or fatal. Adequate dietary zinc, Vitamin C and iron for hemoglobin are also necessary to promote healing.

Guaifenesin

Brand Name: Robitussin®

Category Of Drug: Phlegm Loosener

Intended Effects: To loosen phlegm associated with allergies and respiratory infections.

Side Effects: Side effects are usually mild. Cough medicines which contain guaifenesin and additives may cause nausea, drowsiness, vomiting, dry mouth, nervousness, restlessness, insomnia or headache.

Warnings: Should be used with caution by people with glaucoma or enlarged prostate. Children under the age of 2 should use this drug only as directed by physician. Should be used with caution by people with high blood pressure, heart disorders, diabetes. Should be avoided by people with severe high blood pressure, overactive thyroid, or people taking MAO inhibitors.

Possible Interactions: Risk of bleeding may be increased if this drug is taken with anticlotting drugs like warfarin or heparin.

Note: Some guaifenesin-combination cough medicines are available without Rx prescription.

Guanadrel

Brand Name: Hylorel®

Category Of Drug: Blood-Pressure Reducer

Intended Effects: To treat high blood pressure in people who have not responded to thiazide diuretics.

Side Effects: Faintness, dizziness, weakness, shortness of breath, tiredness, tingling sensations, drowsiness, headache, visual disturbances, increased bowel movements, diarrhea, constipation, frequent or difficult urination, backache, neck ache, ejaculatory failure, impotence, extremely low blood pressure, fluid or salt retention, indigestion, chest pain, loss of appetite, coughing, awareness of heartbeat, confusion, dry mouth, dry throat, gas pain, aching limbs, leg cramps, depression, sleeping problems, nausea, vomiting, weight gain or loss.

Warnings: Do not use in people with history of congestive heart failure. Use with caution in people with vascular disease, bronchial asthma, kidney failure or peptic ulcer. If dizziness or weakness occurs, lie down or sit down to avoid total loss of consciousness. Avoid prolonged standing or exercise, hot weather, alcohol or overheating. Discontinue use at least 72 hours before surgery.

Possible Interactions: Antidepressants, ephedrine, phenylpropanolamine, or phenothiazines can reverse its effects. Ingredients in many over-the-counter medications may interact with this drug — use with caution. Alcohol can increase its effects. Guanadrel may increase the effects of norepinephrine. Beta-blockers, certain blood-pressure regulators, or reserpine may increase its effects. Should not be used within one week of using MAO inhibitors.

Guanethidine

Brand Name: Ismelin®

Category Of Drug: Blood-Pressure Reducer

Intended Effects: To treat moderate to severe high blood pressure.
Side Effects: Dizziness, weakness, tiredness, fainting, diarrhea, fluid retention. Less frequent: fatigue, nausea, vomiting, scalp hair loss, dry mouth, muscle tremor, mental

depression, chest pains, nasal congestion, weight gain, asthma, anemia, blurred vision.

Warnings: Use with caution in patients with kidney disease, heart disease, congestive heart failure, peptic ulcer. Dosage may be reduced in presence of fever. Use with caution in patients with bronchial asthma, since this drug may aggravate that condition.

Possible Interactions: Appetite suppressants, stimulants, oral contraceptives, and tricyclic antidepressants may cause reduced effects. Dosage should be increased gradually if diuretics are being taken. Thiazide diuretics increase the effects of this drug. MAO inhibitor therapy should be stopped 14 days before this medicine is taken.

Gyne-Lotrimin® (*Schering*)
  See: Clotrimazole-Topical

Halcinonide
  See: Adrenocorticoid Class-Topical

Halcion® (*Upjohn*)
  See: Triazolam

Haldol® (*McNeil*)
  See: Haloperidol

Halog® (*Squibb*)

See: Adrenocorticoid Class-Topical

Haloperidol

Brand Name: Haldol®

Category Of Drug: Tranquilizer

Intended Effects: To treat psychotic disorders, hyperactivity and severe behavior problems in children. To control the tics and vocal sounds of Gilles de la Tourette's Syndrome.

Side Effects: Uncontrolled muscle movements and other neuro-muscular reactions; irreversible, involuntary movements of tongue, face, mouth or jaw; insomnia, restlessness, anxiety, elevated mood, aggitation, drowsiness, depression, tiredness, headache, confusion, incoordinated movements, epileptic seizures, hallucinations, rapid heartbeat, low blood pressure, low white blood cell count, anemia and other blood disorders, jaundice and impaired liver function, loss of hair, light-sensitive rashes, skin eruptions, flow of milk from the nipples, enlarged breasts, menstrual irregularities, impotence, change in sex drive, elevated blood sugar or low blood sugar, loss of appetite, constipation, diarrhea, excessive salivation, upset stomach, vomiting, dry mouth, blurred vision, urinary retention, loss of voice, pain in the upper respiratory tract, excessively deep breathing, sudden death.

Warnings: Should not be used in severe, toxic central nervous system depression or coma. Should not be used by people who are sensitive to this drug or to other major tranquilizers or by those who have Parkinson's disease.

Pneumonia may occur in some cases, possibly as a result of dehydration produced by decreased sensation of thirst. Should be used with caution by people with heart disease or high blood pressure. Should be used cautiously by people who have had breast cancer, since it raises prolactin levels which may promote the development of the disease. Causes birth defects in animals — avoid during first three months of pregnancy. Possibly present in mothers' milk — avoid drug or avoid nursing. Should be used with caution by people with glaucoma, epilepsy, high blood pressure, heart disease, impaired kidney or liver function or diseases of these organs. Avoid alcohol completely because of possible increased effects. Should be used with caution by people with allergies. Drive with caution since this drug may cause drowsiness.

Possible Interactions: Sedation may increase when taken with: tranquilizers, antihistamines, antidepressants, sedatives, sleep inducers, alcohol and narcotics. May interfere with anticlotting drugs and levodopa. May interact with blood-pressure reducers to cause excessive lowering of blood pressure. May increase the effects of atropine. May increase the rate of seizures in people taking anticonvulsants. May be poisonous if taken in combination with lithium.

Haltran® (*Upjohn*)
  See: Ibuprofen

Hexachlorophene

Brand Name: pHisoHex®

Category Of Drug: Antibacterial

Intended Effects: To treat bacterial infections of theskin.

Side Effects: Redness, drying or scaling of the skin.

Warnings: For external use only. Any hexachlorophene suds which accidentally get into the eyes while washing should be promptly and thoroughly rinsed out with water. Not for use on burned or denuded skin, mucous membranes in the mouth or genitals, or for total body bathing. Rinse thoroughly after use, especially from sensitive areas such as the genitals. Should be discontinued if signs of irritability occur. Should not be used to wash babies; absorption through the thin skin of infants may cause convulsions and brain damage.

Hycodan® (*Du Pont*)

Category Of Drug: Narcotic, Anticough

Ingredients: Hydrocodone + Homatropine

Intended Effects: To control coughing.

Side Effects: Sedation, nausea, vomiting, constipation.

Warnings: Not for people with glaucoma. Contains a derivative of codeine and can become habit forming. Drug dependence may result from long-term use of high doses. Drive and operate machinery with caution if drowsiness develops.

Possible Interactions: Sedation may increase when taken with: tranquilizers, antihistamines, antidepressants, sedatives, sleep inducers, alcohol and narcotics. May cause depression of brain function when taken with phenytoin.

Hycomine® Syrup (*Du Pont*)

Category Of Drug: Anticough, Decongestant, Narcotic

Ingredients: Hydrocodone + Phenylpropanolamine

Intended Effects: To relieve coughing and nasal congestion.

Side Effects: Drowsiness (especially in children), dizziness, pounding heartbeat, upset stomach, nervousness.

Warnings: Use with caution by people with diabetes, overactive thyroid, high blood pressure, and heart disease. Drive and operate machinery with caution. Use alcohol with extreme caution. Causes birth defects in animals — avoid during first three months of pregnancy. For short term use only — this drug may be habit forming.

Possible Interactions: Sedation may increase when taken with: tranquilizers, antihistamines, antidepressants, sedatives, sleep inducers, alcohol and narcotics.

Hycomine® Tablet (*Du Pont*)

Category Of Drug: Narcotic, Anticough, Pain Reliever, Antihistamine, Decongestant

Ingredients: Hydrocodone + Chlorpheniramine + Phenylephrine + Acetaminophen + Caffeine

Intended Effects: To control coughing, nasal congestion, and congestion in the upper respiratory tract.

Side Effects: Drowsiness, blurred vision, rapid heartbeat, dryness of the mouth, nervousness, dizziness, upset stomach.

Warnings: Not for people who are allergic to any of the ingredients of this drug. Drive and operate machinery with caution because of possible drowsiness or blurred vision. Use with caution by people with high blood pressure, heart disease, overactive thyroid, and advanced age. Causes birth defects in animals — avoid during first three months of pregnancy. For short term use only — this drug may be habit forming.

Possible Interactions: Sedation may increase when taken with: tranquilizers, antihistamines, antidepressants, sedatives, sleep inducers, alcohol and narcotics.

Hydergine® (*Sandoz*)
See: Ergot Mesylates

Hydralazine

Brand Name: Apresoline®

Category Of Drug: Blood-Pressure Reducer

Intended Effects: To lower blood pressure, to increase heart rate, to increase blood flow from the heart, to the kidneys and the brain.

Side Effects: Headache, loss of appetite, nausea, vomiting, diarrhea, aggravation of angina pectoris, nasal congestion, numbness or tingling of hands or feet, fluid retention, dizziness, muscle cramps or tremors, depression or anxiety, rash, chills, fever, constipation, difficulty in urination, anemia, reduction in red blood count, joint aches, swelling of feet, irregular heartbeat, watery eyes.

Warnings: Should not be taken by patients with certain serious heart or kidney diseases. Causes birth defects in animals — avoid during first three months of pregnancy Known to be present in mothers' milk — avoid drug or avoid nursing. Complete blood count tests should be done before and during treatment.

Possible Interactions: MAO inhibitor antidepressants should be given with caution to patients on this drug. May increase action of other blood-pressure reducers. The effects of alcohol and other non-prescription drugs may be increased. Antihistamines may reduce its effectiveness. Heavy exercise and exposure to cold may increase this drug's tendency to cause angina in certain individuals. Diuretics may increase its effects.

Hydrochlorothiazide
See: Thiazide Diuretic Class

Hydrocortisone
See: Adrenocorticoid Class

HydroDiuril® (*Merck Sharp & Dohme*)

See: Thiazide Diuretic Class

Hydroflumethiazide
See: Thiazide Diuretic Class

Hydropres® (*Merck Sharp & Dohme*)
See: Rauwolfia Alkaloid Class
See: Thiazide Diuretic Class

Hydroxyzine

Brand Names: Atarax®, Vistaril®

Category Of Drug: Tranquilizer, Antihistamine

Intended Effects: To restore emotional calmness; to relieve anxiety, apprehension, agitation, tension.

Side Effects: Drowsiness, itching, headache, dryness of mouth.

Warnings: Use caution when driving or operating machinery. Use alcohol with extreme caution. Causes birth defects in animals – avoid during first three months of pregnancy and use with extreme caution during last six months. Known to be present in mothers' milk – avoid drug or avoid nursing.

Possible Interactions: Hydroxyzine may increase the effects of anticlotting drugs: (acenocoumarol, dicumarol, phenprocoumon, warfarin). May decrease the effects of phenytoin (Dilantin®). Sedation may increase when taken with: tranquilizers, antihistamines, antidepressants, sedatives, sleep inducers, alcohol and narcotics.

Hygroton® (*USV*)
See: Thiazide Diuretic Class

Note: Its chemical structure is slightly different than thiazides, but its effects are similar.

Hylorel® (*Pennwalt*)
See: Guanadrel

Hytone® (*Dermik*)
See: Adrenocorticoid Class-Topical

Iberet-Folic-500® (*Abbott*)
See: Fero-Folic-500

Ibuprofen

Brand Names: Prescription Only — Motrin®, Rufen®
Over-The Counter — Advil®, Haltran®, Medipren®, Nuprin®, Trendar®

Category Of Drug: Anti-inflammatory, Pain Reliever, Fever Reducer

Intended Effects: To reduce inflammation in cases of

rheumatoid and osteoarthritis. To reduce joint swelling, pain, stiffness, to increase movement; to relieve menstrual cramps.

Side Effects: Frequent (4-16%): nausea, stomach pain, heartburn, diarrhea, vomiting, indigestion, constipation, abdominal cramps or pain, bloating, gas. Less frequent (1-3%): dizziness, headache, nervousness, rash, ringing in the ears, increased appetite, fluid retention. Infrequent (less than 1%): stomach or duodenal ulcers, skin eruptions, depression, insomnia, visual disturbances, blood disorders, congestive heart failure in people with poor heart function, elevated blood pressure. Rare (reported but unconfirmed): hepatitis, jaundice, abnormal liver function, tingling sensations, hallucinations, loss of hair, infection of the eyes, double vision, pain in the eyes, rare blood disorders, fever low blood sugar, interruption of heart rhythm, impaired kidney function.

Warnings: Safety of this drug for children has not been determined. Not for people who are allergic to any dosage of this drug or to aspirin. Should be used with great caution by people with upper gastrointestinal tract disease, people taking anticlotting drugs, or people with history of ulcers or poor heart function. Bleeding time may be prolonged while taking this medicine.

Possible Interactions: Combined stomach lining irritation from alcohol and irritant action of this drug in sensitive individuals can increase the risk of stomach ulceration or bleeding in sensitive people. Combined use of this drug and aspirin is not recommended. May increase the chance of bleeding when given with anticlotting drugs. Works against the effectiveness of diuretics, so it may contribute to lack of effectiveness of these drugs in people taking both diuretics and ibuprofen. Fluid retention can be minimized by a salt-restricted diet.

Iletin® (*Lilly*)
See: Insulin

Ilosone® (*Dista*)
See: Erythromycin Class

Imipramine
See: Tricyclic Antidepressant Class

Imodium® (*Janssen*)
See: Loperamide

Inderal® (*Ayerst*)
See: Beta-Adrenergic Blocking Agent Class

Inderide® (*Ayerst*)
See: Thiazide Diuretic Class
See: Beta-Adrenergic Blocking Agent Class

Indocin® (*Merck Sharp & Dohme*)
See: Indomethacin

Indomethacin

Brand Name: Indocin®

Category Of Drug: Anti-inflammatory, Fever Reducer, Pain Reliever.

Intended Effects: To relieve pain and inflammation in arthritis and similar conditions which have not responded to treatment with aspirin or other salicylates.

Side Effects: Frequent (more than 1%): nausea, vomiting, upset stomach, diarrhea, abdominal pain or distress, constipation, headache, dizziness, vertigo, sleepiness, depression, fatigue, listlessness, ringing in the ears. Less frequent (less than 1%): loss of appetite, bloating, passing gas, peptic ulcer, intestinal problems, bleeding from the rectum, inflammation of the prostate, ulcers, perforation and bleeding from the esophagus, stomach, duodenum or small intestine. Rare: gastro-intestinal bleeding without obvious ulcers, hepatitis, jaundice, anxiety, muscle weakness, involuntary muscle movements, insomnia, mental disorders, drowsiness, lightheadedness, blackouts, tingling sensations, increased symptoms of epilepsy and Parkinson's disease in people who have those conditions, coma, convulsions, blurred vision, hearing disturbances, deafness, deposits in the cornea and retina of the eye, high blood pressure, disturbances in heartbeat, chest pain, fluid retention, weight gain, reddening or flushing of the skin, sweating, elevated blood sugar and other blood components, itching, rash, peeling of the skin, loss of hair, low white blood cell count, bone marrow depression, anemia, bleeding under the skin, difficult breathing, shock, hive-like rash, asthma, bleeding from the urogenital tract.

Warnings: Not for children under 14. Should be used with caution by the elderly, and by those with epilepsy, blood clotting defects, parkinsonism, poor kidney or liver function. Drive and operate machinery with caution, since this drug effects mental alertness and coordination. Should not be taken by people who have allergic reactions to aspirin or other non-adrenocorticoid anti-inflammatory drugs. Should not be used by people who have nasal polyps associated with angioedema, a hive-like allergic reaction. Should not be taken by people who have a history of ulcers or other lesions in the gastro-intestinal tract. The side effects from taking indomethacin are dosage related, so the lowest effective dose should be used. May mask usual signs of infection. Known to be present in mothers' milk — avoid drug or avoid nursing.

Possible Interactions: Aspirin decreases the blood levels of indomethacin slightly, and probenecid increases blood levels of indomethacin. Lithium concentration may rise while taking indomethacin, so close monitoring is advised by people taking lithium. Indomethacin may interfere with the blood pressure reducing effects of furosemide.

Insulin

Category Of Drug: Pancreatic Hormone, Antidiabetic

Intended Effects: To control diabetes, to lower blood sugar and restore the body's ability to use sugar normally.

Side Effects: Symptoms of high blood sugar (hyperglycemia) indicating that insulin requirements may be greater than what is currently being supplied are: increased urination, loss of appetite, thirst, bad breath, dry skin. Symptoms of low blood sugar (hypoglycemia), indicating that the body may have too much insulin available are: rapid pulse, shakiness, tiredness, weakness, shock, chills, cold sweat, drowsiness, hunger, headache.

Warnings: When people take more insulin than they require, symptoms of low blood sugar (hypoglycemia) may be eliminated by quickly eating a sugary food like a candy bar to keep the symptoms from worsening and possibly leading to insulin shock. Avoid alcohol or use with caution. Insulin dose, schedule and diet require careful control and monitoring by both patient and physician. Insulin dose may need changing for those with kidney or liver impairment, overactive or underactive thyroid, nausea or vomiting, surgery, high fever or during pregnancy. Periods of heavy exercise and missing meals may lead to low blood sugar.

Possible Interactions: MAO inhibitors or large doses of salicylates may increase the blood-sugar-lowering effect. Adrenal hormones, thiazide or thiazide-related diuretics, thyroid hormones and epinephrine may increase the possibility of high blood sugar.

Ionamin® (*Pennwalt*)
  See: Appetite Suppressant Class

Iron Supplements
  See: Ferrous Sulfate

Ismelin® (*CIBA*)
  See: Guanethidine

Isoclor® (*American Critical Care*)

See: Antihistamine Class
See: Pseudoephedrine

Isoetharine

Brand Names: Bronkometer®, Bronkosol®

Category Of Drug: Bronchial-Tube Relaxer

Intended Effects: To open lung passages in bronchial asthma, bronchitis and emphysema by inhalation.

Side Effects: Frequent use may cause nausea, headache, changes in blood pressure, tension, restlessness, insomnia, weakness, dizziness, excitement, pounding heartbeat, anxiety.

Warnings: May lose effectiveness with excessive use. Should be used with caution by people with high blood pressure, overactive thyroid, or heart disease. Physician should be consulted immediately if breathing difficulty worsens with use.

Possible Interactions: Should not be taken with epinephrine or other direct heart stimulants.

Isoptin® (*Knoll*)
See: Calcium Channel Inhibitor Class

Isopto Carpine® (*Alcon*)
See: Pilocarpine

Isordil® *(Wyeth)*
See: Nitrate Class

Isosorbide Dinitrate
See: Nitrate Class

Isotretinoin

Category Of Drug: Vitamin/Mineral Supplement

Intended Effects: To treat severe cystic acne.

Side Effects: Dry skin, dry nose and mouth, swollen lips, pink eye, itching, nosebleeds, hair loss, extra tissue growth during healing, drying of mucous membranes, nail brittleness, nausea, vomiting, abdominal pain, rash, increase in acne flare-ups including bleeding, puss and skin granules, skin inflammation, peeling palms and soles, skin infections, sensitivity to sun, swelling around fingernails and toenails, increase in blood fats (triglycerides, cholesterol, and lipids), decrease in HDL levels, headaches, visual disturbances, false brain tumor symptoms, tender stiff or painful joints, bones or muscles, high blood calcium concentrations, abnormal liver function, hives, prickly skin sensations, mental depression, weight loss, tiredness, mild bleeding, bruising, and water retention.

Warnings: Causes severe birth defects — avoid during pregnancy. Should be avoided by women of childbearing potential if not using effective contraception. May be present in mothers' milk — avoid drug or avoid nursing. Accutane® should be taken with food, or one hour before or after a meal. Use with caution in diabetics, overweight people, those who consume high amounts of alcohol, or people sensitive to parabens (which is used as a preservative). Avoid long exposure to sunlight.

Possible Interactions: Avoid Vitamin A supplements which may cause increased side effects. Use with caution with tetracycline or minocycline. Minimize or eliminate alcohol intake.

Isoxsuprine

Brand Name: Vasodilan®

Category Of Drug: Blood-Vessel Enlarger

Intended Effects: To relieve symptoms associated with insufficient blood circulation to the brain and other areas of the body, as in Buerger's disease, Raynaud's disease, arteriosclerosis obliterans, or thromboangiitis obliterans.

Side Effects: Low blood pressure, rapid heartbeat, nausea, vomiting, dizziness, abdominal distress, rash.

Warnings: Should not be given immediately after birth or in the presence of arterial bleeding. Should not be given by injection in cases of low blood pressure or rapid heartbeat.

Isuprel® Mistometer (*Breon*)

Category Of Drug: Bronchial-Tube Relaxer

Ingredient: Isoproterenol

Intended Effects: To relieve difficult breathing associated with bronchial asthma, bronchitis and emphysema.

Side Effects: Nervousness, nausea, vomiting, rapid or irregular heartbeat. Rare: headache, tremor, dizziness, sweating, flushing of the skin, weakness, pain in chest or radiating down left arm.

Warnings: Not for people with irregular heartbeat. Should be used with caution by patients with diabetes, overactive thyroid, heart disease, high blood pressure. Avoid excessive use, since this drug loses its effectiveness if overused. Causes birth defects in animals — avoid during first three months of pregnancy. Use caution while driving or operating machinery if dizziness or nervousness occurs.

Possible Interactions: Allow at least four hours between using this drug and epinephrine to avoid serious disturbances of heart rhythm. Should not be taken within 14 days of MAO inhibitor drugs. Propranolol may decrease its effects. Antidepressants and isoproterenol may increase each other's effects.

Kaon® (*Adria*)
  See: Potassium Supplement Class

Kay Ciel® (*Berlex*)
  See: Potassium Supplement Class

Keflex® (*Dista*)
  See: Cephalosporin Class

Kenalog® (*Squibb*)

See: Adrenocorticoid Class - Systemic
See: Adrenocorticoid Class-Topical

Kenalog® in Orabase® (*Squibb*)

Category Of Drug: Anti-inflammatory, Anti-itching, Anti-allergy

Ingredients: Triamcinolone + an emollient dental paste (gelatin, pectin, carboxymethylcellulose, mineral oil, and a polyethylene).

Intended Effects: To provide temporary relief to ulcers, sores or injuries in the mouth or on the gums.

Side Effects: Prolonged use may cause reactions common to other topical steroid reactions: burning, itching, irritation, dryness, slight infection.

Warnings: If irritation worsens or does not improve within a week, consult your physician. Should not be used if any type of infection (fungal, bacterial or viral) is present in mouth or throat. Should not be used by patients with tuberculosis, peptic ulcer or diabetes.

Ketoprofen

Brand Name: Orudis®

Category Of Drug: Anti-inflammatory, Pain Reliever, Fever Reducer, Anti-arthritic

Intended Effects: To reduce inflammation in cases of rheumatoid and osteoarthritis.

Side Effects: Frequent (1-11%): indigestion, nausea, abdominal pain, diarrhea, constipation, flatulence, loss of appetite, vomiting, inflammation of the mucous lining of the mouth, headache, dizziness, ringing in the ears, visual disturbances, rash, water retention, abnormal liver function, irritated urinary tract. Infrequent (less than 1%): increased appetite, dry mouth, belching, inflammation of the lining of the stomach, bleeding from the rectum, black and tarry stools, blood in stools, salivation, peptic ulcer, intestinal ulcer, vomiting blood, loss of memory, confusion, impotence, migraine, tingling sensations, loss of balance, pink eye, eye pain, hearing impairment, change in taste, loss of hair, inflammation of the skin, itching, sweating, hives, sensitivity to the sun, skin discoloration, nails separating from the skin, chills, facial swelling, infection, pain, allergic reaction, anaphylaxis, high blood pressure, awareness of heartbeat, increased heart rate, heart failure, blood vessel problems, enlarged blood vessels, lowered ability of the blood to clot, blood disorders, thirst, weight gain, weight loss, kidney problems, muscle pain, difficult breathing, coughing up of blood, nosebleed, inflammation of the throat, inflammation of the mucous membrane of the nose, swelling of the larnyx, blood in the urine. Rare (reported but unconfirmed): inflammation of the colon, hallucination, changes in sex drive, nightmares, personality disorder, shock, irregular heartbeat, heart attack, aggravated diabetes, jaundice, enlargement of the breasts in males.

Warnings: Should be taken with antacids, food or drink to reduce stomach irritation. Should be used with great caution by people with gastrointestinal bleeding, peptic ulcers, poor kidney function, low blood hemoglobin, fluid retention, high blood pressure, or history of heart failure. Bleeding-time may be prolonged when taking this medicine. Known to be present in mothers' milk — avoid drug or avoid nursing.

Possible Interactions: Combined use of this drug and aspirin, methotrexate or probenecid is not recommended. May change the effects of thiazide diuretics or warfarin — use together with caution. May increase the bleeding time when taken with anticlotting drugs.

K-Lor® (*Abbott*)
  See: Potassium Supplement Class

Klotrix® (*Mead Johnson*)
  See: Potassium Supplement Class

K-Lyte® (*Mead Johnson*)
  See: Potassium Supplement Class

Konsyl (*Lafayette*)
  See: Laxatives-Bulk Class

Note: No Rx prescription required

K-Tab™ (*Abbott*)
  See: Potassium Supplement Class

Kwell® (*Reed & Carnrick*)
See: Lindane

Labetalol

Brand Names: Normodyne®, Trandate®

Category Of Drug: Blood-Pressure Reducer

Intended Effects: To treat high blood pressure.

Side Effects: Dizziness, nausea, tiredness, loss of strength, headache, indigestion, altered taste, stuffy nose, impotence, ejaculation failure, fluid retention, rash, faintness upon rising, tingling sensations of the scalp, loss of balance, changes in vision, difficult breathing, inflammation of skin and internal organs (systemic lupus erythematosus), dry ees, jaundice, muscle cramps, muscle disease, narrowing of air passages in the lungs, difficult urination, depression, disorientation, memory loss.

Warnings: Should not be used by people with bronchial asthma, colon problems, certain blood disorders or those who have experienced heart failure, blocked arteries or slow heartbeat. Do NOT stop abruptly — medication should be stopped gradually under a doctor's care. Use with extreme caution in people with bronchitis, emphysema, diabetes or poor kidney function. Present in mothers' milk — avoid drug or avoid nursing. Safety in children has not been established.

Possible Interactions: Cimetidine increases labetalol's effectiveness. May affect anesthesia required during surgery; larger doses of bronchial tube relaxers may be required. May cause tremors when taken with tricyclic antidepressants. Insulin requirements for diabetics may need to be adjusted. Labetalol reduces effects of nitroglycerin.

Lanoxin® (*Burroughs Wellcome*)
  See: Digitalis Class

Larotid® (*Roche*)
  See: Penicillin Class

Lasix® (*Hoechst-Roussel*)
  See: Furosemide

Laxative-Bulk Class

Generic/Brand Names:
  Psyllium/ Effersyllium®, Konsyl®, Metamucil®,
  Serutan®

Category Of Drug: Laxative-Bulk

Intended Effects: To promote bowel movements by adyding bulk and retaining water in the stool, thus softening stools; to aid in treating spastic or irritable colon or hemorrhoids; to reduce straining with senility and heart problems; to regulate bowel movements during pregnancy.

Side Effects: Pink coloration of urine (harmless). Rare: asthma, skin rash, itching, swallowing difficulty, intestinal blockage.

171

Warnings: While taking this medicine, drink plenty of liquids for proper effect and to avoid blocking the intestine. Should be used with caution by people on low-calorie, low-salt or low-sugar diets. Not for use if signs of appendicitis or inflamed bowels are present. Should be used with caution by people with diabetes, high blood pressure, heart disease, colostomy or ileostomy, kidney disease, intestinal blockage.

Note: No Rx prescription required

Laxative-Emollient Class

Brand Names: Colace®, Surfak®

Category Of Drug: Laxative-emollient

Intended Effects: To promote bowel movements by helping liquids mix into the stools.

Side Effects: Harmless discoloration of urine, bitter taste, stomach cramps, throat irritation, skin rash, itching.

Warnings: Considered safe for pregnant and nursing women. Should not be taken if vomiting, abdominal pain, nausea, or signs of appendicitis or inflamed bowel are present. Not all emollient laxatives are acceptable for children — consult physician for guidance. Should not be taken within two hours of other medicine because it may reduce the effects of the other medicine. Do not take with mineral oil.

Note: No Rx prescription required

Laxative-Hyperosmotic Class

Generic Name: Epsom Salts

Category Of Drug: Laxative-hyperosmotic

Intended Effects: To promote bowel movements by bringing water into the bowel from surrounding body tissues.

Side Effects: Stomach or intestinal cramps, throat irritation with liquid form of this medicine. Rare: skin rash, dizziness, irregular heartbeat, mental confusion, unusual tiredness, unpleasant taste which may be relieved by drinking citrus juice after each dose.

Warnings: Laxatives are more effective if large amounts of liquid are also taken. Should be used with caution by people with high blood pressure, diabetes, congestive heart disease, colostomy or ileostomy, kidney disease, ulcerative colitis, or those people showing signs of appendicitis. Not for children under the age of 6 unless prescribed by physician. If taken within two hours of other medicines, effects of the other medicine may be reduced. Not for people who need a low galactose diet. Not for treatment longer than one-week. Long-term use may result in dependence.

Possible Interactions: May reduce the effects of tetracycline antibiotics. This type of laxative may contain large amounts of sugar or salt, which may alter the effectiveness of antidiabetic drugs and blood-pressure reducers.

Note: No Rx prescription required

Laxative-Lubricant Class

Generic Name: Mineral Oil

Category Of Drug: Laxative-lubricant

Intended Effects: To promote bowel movements by coating the stool and bowel with a waterproof film.

Side Effects: Usually none if directions are followed and dose is not exceeded.

Warnings: Not for children under the age of six. Should be used with caution by people with diabetes, heart disease, ileostomy or colostomy or signs of appendicitis. Laxatives are more effective if large amounts of water are also consumed. Should not be taken within two hours of eating because of possible interference with digestion of food. Avoid during pregnancy. For short-term use only. Do not take with stool softeners. Prolonged use can lead to deficiency of fat soluble vitamins like vitamin A.

Possible Interactions: Lubricant laxatives should not be taken within two hours of other medicines, especially birth control pills or anticlotting drugs, to avoid reducing the effect of the other medicines.

Note: No Rx prescription required

Laxative-Stimulant Class

Generic/Brand Names:
  Bisacodyl/Dulcolax®

Danthron/Modane®
Phenolphthalein/Ex-Lax®
Senna/Senokot®

Category Of Drug: Laxative-stimulant

Intended Effects: To encourage bowel movements by increasing muscle contractions.

Side Effects: Belching, cramping, nausea, diarrhea, unpleasant taste, skin rash. Notify physician if irregular heartbeat, breathing difficulty, confusion, skin rash or unusual tiredness occurs from taking this drug. Occasional insignificant discoloration of urine or stool (red or pink).

Warnings: Not for people who have had reactions to laxatives in the past. Works best when taken on an empty stomach. Do not take this laxative if you have abdominal pains. Not for treatment of more than one week. If taken within two hours of another medicine, the effects of the other medicine may be reduced. Stimulant laxatives, should be avoided by pregnant women since they may cause unwanted effects such as contractions of the womb. May be present in mothers' milk — avoid drug or avoid nursing. Long-term and frequent use may result in dependence.

Possible Interactions: Do not take within two hours of other medicines because it may decrease the effects of the other medicine. Do not take with mineral oil.

Note: No Rx prescription required

Ledercillin® VK (*Lederle*)
See: Penicillin Class

Levothroid® (*USV*)
See: Thyroid Hormone   Class

Levothyroxine
See: Thyroid Hormone Class

Librax® (*Roche*)

Category Of Drug: Tranquilizer

Ingredients: Chlordiazepoxide + Clidinium

Intended Effects: To control emotional and body factors in gastrointestinal disorders like peptic ulcer, irritable bowel, and enterocolitis.

Side Effects: Drowsiness, incoordinated movements, confusion, skin rashes, retention of fluid and swelling, menstrual irregularities, reduced milk production, changes in sexual desire, blood and liver disorders, dryness of the mouth, blurring of vision, difficult urination, constipation, unsteadiness in standing or walking, fainting, blurred vision, dizziness, nausea.

Warnings: Not for patients with glaucoma, enlargement of the prostate, bladder neck obstruction. Drive and operate machinery with caution. Librax® is habit-forming, and physical and psychological dependence can result. Withdrawal symptoms may include nervousness, tremor, and convulsions. Suicidal tendencies may come to the surface in depressed patients. Use with caution in patients with impaired kidney or liver function. May cause birth defects —

avoid during first three months of pregnancy. Known to be present in mothers' milk — avoid drug or avoid nursing.

Possible Interactions: Sedation may increase when taken with: tranquilizers, antihistamines, antidepressants, sedatives, sleep inducers, alcohol and narcotics. If taken with MAO inhibitors, extreme sedation and convulsions may occur.

Librium® *(Roche)*
  See: Benzodiazepine Class

Lidex® *(Syntex)*
  See: Adrenocorticoid Class-Topical

Limbitrol® *(Roche)*
  See: Benzodiazepine Class
  See: Tricyclic Antidepressant Class

Lindane

Brand Name: Kwell®

Category Of Drug: Antiparasite

Ingredients: Gamma Benzene Hexachloride

Intended Effects: Applied directly to the skin to kill skin and scalp parasites such as scabies, head lice, crab lice and their eggs.

Side Effects: Skin rashes.

Warnings: Should be used with caution by pregnant women, children and infants. Do not exceed recommended dose. Harmful to the brain — seizures have been reported from excessive absorption of this drug through the skin. Flush eyes with water if this medicine accidentally contacts eyes. Avoid simultaneous application of creams, ointments or oils which may enhance absorption.

Liothyronine
See: Thyroid Hormone Class

Liotrix
See: Thyroid Hormone Class

Lithium

Brand Name: Eskalith®

Category Of Drug: Tranquilizer

Intended Effects: To treat manic episodes of manic-depressive mental illness.

Side Effects: Increased thirst, hand tremor, lethargy, drowsiness, itching, headache, blurred vision, slurred speech, dizziness, restlessness, stupor, confusion, diarrhea, vomiting.

Warnings: Patient should consult physician if diarrhea, vomiting, drowsiness, muscular weakness or tremor occur since this may indicate lithium buildup to poisonous levels. Physical and mental abilities may be lowered — drive and operate machinery with caution. Known to be present in-mothers' milk — avoid drug or avoid nursing. May cause birth defects. Avoid during first three months of pregnancy. Not for children under the age of 12. Not for people taking diuretics, those with severe heart or kidney disease, those who are severely dehydrated. People taking lithium should also have an adequate salt intake in their diet. Use alcohol with extreme caution. Dosage of this drug must be carefully regulated to avoid drug poisoning. Goiters may develop with long-term use.

Possible Interactions: If haloperidol and lithium are taken together, blood tests should be monitored closely to avoid poisoning. Other antipsychotic drugs may reduce the effectiveness of this drug. Lithium may prolong the effects of drugs affecting the nervous system and muscle system. Diuretics taken with lithium may cause severe lithium poisoning because of excessive loss of sodium and retention of lithium.

Lithostat™ (*Mission*)
  See: Acetohydroxamic Acid

Loestrin® (*Parke-Davis*)
  See: Estrogen + Progestin   Class

Loestrin® **FE** (*Parke-Davis*)
  See: Estrogen +   Progestin Class

Note: Same as Loestrin®, plus brown tablets which are

iron supplements.

Lomotil® (*Searle*)

Category Of Drug: Antidiarrhea

Ingredients: Diphenoxylate + Atropine

Intended Effects: To control diarrhea and to relieve intestinal cramps.

Side Effects: Dry skin and mouth, flushing, fever, interruptions of heart rhythm, urinary retention, loss of appetite, nausea, vomiting, abdominal discomfort, intestinal blockage, toxic colon, itching, swelling of gums, rashes, retention of fluid, dizziness, drowsiness, sedation, headache, lethargy, restlessness, euphoria, depression, coma, tingling sensations.

Warnings: Should be used with caution in children. While combating the symptoms it may increase the damage done by micro-organisms in cases of diarrhea. Should be used with extreme caution in people with ulcerative colitis, liver or kidney disease. Addiction and drug dependence can result if extremely high doses are taken, but not at the recommended doses.

Possible Interactions: Sedation may increase when taken with: tranquilizers, antihistamines, antidepressants, sedatives, sleep inducers, alcohol and narcotics. If taken with MAO inhibitors, excessive rise in blood pressure may result.

Lo/Ovral® (*Wyeth*)

See: Estrogen and Progestin Class

Loperamide

Brand Name: Imodium®

Category Of Drug: Antidiarrhea

Intended Effects: To control diarrhea; to reduce discharge from ileostomies.

Side Effects: Stomach pain or bloatedness, constipation, drowsiness, dizziness, dry mouth, nausea, vomiting, tiredness, skin rash.

Warnings: Should not be used by people who should not be subjected to constipation. Should be used cautiously by patients with liver disease or colitis. Notify your doctor if diarrhea continues 48 hours after beginning this medication or if fever develops. Not for children under 12.

Possible Interactions: Since diarrhea can cause severe loss of fluids and electrolytes, extra intake of fluids is advised even when this medication is taken.

Lopressor® (*Geigy*)
See: Beta-Adrenergic Blocking Agent

Lopressor HCT® (*Geigy*)

Category Of Drug: Blood-Pressure Reducer, Diuretic

Ingredients: Metoprolol + Hydrochlorothiazide

Intended Effects: To reduce blood pressure, to slow and strengthen heartbeat, to regulate irregular heartbeat, to eliminate excess fluid from the body.

Note: This is a combination of a beta blocker (Metoprolol) and a thiazide diuretic (Hydrochlorothiazide).

See: Beta-Adrenergic Blocking Agent Class
See: Thiazide Diuretic Class

Lopurin® (*Boots*)
  See: Allopurinol

Lorazepam
  See: Benzodiazepine Class

Lotrimin® (*Schering*)
  See: Clotrimazole-Topical

Ludiomil® (*CIBA*)
  See: Maprotiline

Lufyllin® (*Wallace*)
  See: Xanthine Class

Lufyllin®-GG (*Wallace*)

See: Guaifenesin
See: Xanthine Class

Luride® (*Colgate-Hoyt Laboratories*)
See:Fluoride

Maalox® (*Rorer*)

Category Of Drug: Antacid

Ingredients: Magnesium + Aluminum Hydroxide

Intended Effects: To relieve heartburn or acid indigestion, and to relieve discomfort associated with ulcers, gastritis and hernias without causing constipation.

Warnings: Do not exceed recommended dosage. Do not take maximum dosage for longer than two weeks. Do not use this drug if you have kidney disease, except under the supervision of physician. Not for use by children.

Possible Interactions: Decreases the effects of tetracycline and phenytoin.

Note: No Rx prescription required

Macrodantin® (*Norwich Eaton*)
See: Nitrofurantoin Macrocrystals

Mandelamine® (*Parke-Davis*)
See: Methenamine Mandelate

MAO Inhibitors
See: Monoamine Oxidase Inhibitor Class

Maprotiline

Brand Name: Ludiomil®

Category Of Drug: Tricyclic Antidepressant

Intended Effects: To treat depressive illnesses such as depressive neurosis, manic-depressive illness, depressed type, and to relieve anxiety associated with depression.

Side Effects: Dry mouth, constipation, blurred vision, skin rash, pounding, irregular or rapid heartbeat, drowsiness, dizziness, tremor, nausea, weakness, fatigue, headache.

Warnings: Not for people recovering from recent heart attack, those who are allergic to this drug, or those with known or suspected seizure disorders. Should be used with caution by people with heart disease, over active thyroid, glaucoma, history of urinary retention, increased pressure within the eye. Drive and operate machinery with caution since this drug may impair alertness. This drug should be discontinued for as long as possible before elective surgery.

Possible Interactions: Should not be given within 14 days of MAO inhibitors. If given with nervous-system regulators or sympathomimetic drugs, additive atropine-like effects may result. Thyroid medication may increase the possibility of cardiovascular toxicity of Ludiomil®. May block the beneficial effects of guanethidine. Sedation may increase when taken with: tranquilizers, antihistamines, antidepressants, sleep inducers, sedatives, alcohol and narcotics.

Marax® (*Roerig*)

Category Of Drug: Bronchial-Tube Relaxer, Blood-Vessel Narrower

Ingredients: Ephedrine + Theophylline + Hydroxyzine

Intended Effects: To treat and help prevent bronchial asthma, to relieve congestion of breathing passages.

Side Effects: Nervousness, insomnia, headache, drowsiness, chest discomfort, nausea, vomiting, excitation, dryness of the nose and throat, rapid or pounding heartbeat, urinary difficulties.

Warnings: Causes birth defects in animals — avoid during first three months of pregnancy. Known to be present in mothers' milk — avoid drug or avoid nursing. Not for people with high blood pressure, over-active thyroid, or heart disease. Should be used with caution by people with prostate enlargement. Not for children under the age of two. Because of possible drowsiness, drive and operate machinery with caution. Tolerance may develop with large doses over a long time period.

Possible Interactions: Sedation may increase when taken with: tranquilizers, antihistamines, antidepressants, sedatives, sleep inducers, alcohol and narcotics. Many over-the-counter drugs for allergies and colds contain ingredients which may interact with Marax®. May decrease the effects of blood-pressure reducers and increase the effects of epinephrine.

Marax® DF Syrup (*Roerig*)
See: Marax®

Note: This is a pediatric syrup. The DF means dye-free...no coloring which might cause an allergic reaction is added.

Materna® (*Lederle*)

Category Of Drug: Vitamin/Mineral Supplement

Ingredients: Vitamin A + D + E + C + Folic Acid + Thiamine + Riboflavin + Vitamin B6 + Niacinamide + Vitamin B12 + Calcium + Iodine + Elemental Iron + Magnesium + Copper + Zinc

Intended Effects: To provide necessary vitamins and minerals during pregnancy and nursing.

Side Effects: Possible allergic sensitization from the folic acid.

Warnings: Folic acid may obscure results from blood tests for anemia.

Maxitrol® (*Alcon*)

Category Of Drug: Anti-infective

Ingredients: Dexamethasone + Neomycin + Polymyxin B

Intended Effects: To treat inflammation and allergic reactions in the eye or ear.

Side Effects: In the eye: burning, stinging, watering, blurred vision, pain, drooping of the eyelids. In the ear: burning or stinging of the ear, fungus infection. Long term treatment: cataracts or glaucoma.

Warnings: Should be used with great caution by people with herpes simplex, glaucoma, fungus infections in the eye or ear, perforated eardrum, chicken pox or cowpox.

Possible Interactions: When used with adrenal hormones or antibiotics, fungus infections may develop.

Maxzide® (*Lederle*)

Category Of Drug: Blood Pressure Reducer, Diuretic

Ingredients: Triamterene + Hydrochlorothiazide

Intended Effects: To reduce blood pressure, to eliminate excess fluid from the body.

  See: Triamterene
  See: Thiazide Diuretic Class

Mebaral® (*Breon*)
See: Barbiturate Class

Mebendazole

Brand Name: Vermox®

Category Of Drug: Antiparasite

Intended Effects: To destroy and remove parasitic worms such as tapeworms, roundworms, pinworms and hookworms.

Side Effects: Abdominal pain, diarrhea.

Warnings: Causes birth defects in animals — avoid during pregnancy. Use with caution in children under two years.

Meclizine

Brand Names: Antivert®, Ru-Vert 2®

Category Of Drug: Antihistamine

Intended Effects: To relieve nausea and vomiting, to control dizziness associated with motion sickness or inner-ear disturbances.

Side Effects: Drowsiness, dry mouth. Rare: blurred vision.

Warnings: Causes birth defects in animals — avoid during first three months of pregnancy and use with extreme caution during last six months. Because of possible drowsiness, drive and operate machinery with caution. Not recommended for children.

Possible Interactions: Sedation may increase when

taken with: tranquilizers, antihistamines, antidepressants, sedatives, sleep inducers, alcohol and narcotics.

Meclofenamate

Brand Name: Meclomen®

Category Of Drug: Anti-inflammatory, Anti-arthritic

Intended Effects: To relieve the symptoms of rheumatoid arthritis and osteoarthritis.

Side Effects: Most frequent (10-33%): diarrhea, nausea, vomiting, stomach discomfort, abdominal pain, gas. Frequent (3-9%): rash, headache, dizziness, heartburn, loss of appetite. Less frequent (1-3%): ringing in the ears, constipation, peptic ulcer, fluid retention. Rare (reports are unconfirmed): depression, sleeplessness, fatigue, blurred vision, awareness of heartbeat.

Warnings: Causes birth defects in animals — avoid during pregnancy. Should not be used by patients sensitive to this drug or to aspirin. Should be taken cautiously by those with a history of upper gastrointestinal tract disease. Diarrhea should be reported to your doctor; it can usually be controlled by adjusting this drug's dosage. Take with food or antacids to avoid possible stomach distress.

Possible Interactions: Increases the effectiveness of warfarin. Aspirin lowers levels of this drug in the blood; both taken together may cause bloody stools.

Meclomen® (*Parke-Davis*)

See: Meclofenamate

Medipren® (*Johnson & Johnson*)
See: Ibuprofen

Medrol® (*Upjohn*)
  See: Adrenocorticoid Class - Systemic
  See: Adrenocorticoid Class - Topical

Medroxyprogesterone
  See: Progestin Class

Mefenamic Acid

Brand Name: Ponstel®

Category Of Drug: Anti-inflammatory, Pain Reliever, Fever Reducer

Intended Effects: To treat mild to moderate pain.

Side Effects: Nausea, stomach distress, vomiting, gas, and diarrhea which may be severe. Drowsiness, dizziness, nervousness, headache, blurred vision, insomnia, itching, rash, eye irritation, ear pain, perspiration. Rare: reversible loss of color vision, throbbing heartbeat, difficult breathing. With long term use: anemia.

Warnings: Not for people with intestinal infections or for children under 14. Should be used with caution by people with asthma, kidney or liver disease. Known to be present in mothers' milk — avoid drug or avoid nursing. Notify physician if rash or diarrhea occurs since this indicates need to discontinue drug. Take with food or antacids to ease possible stomach discomfort.

Possible Interactions: May increase the effects of anti-clotting drugs. If taken with alcohol or aspirin, risk of stomach or intestinal discomfort is increased. May decrease effectiveness of insulin in diabetics — dose may need to be adjusted.

Mellaril® (*Sandoz*)
  See: Phenothiazine Class

Meperidine

Brand Name: Demerol® Oral

Category Of Drug: Pain Reliever, Narcotic

Intended Effects: To relieve moderate to severe pain; to prepare for anesthesia.

Side Effects: Lightheadedness, dizziness, nausea, sedation, vomiting, sweating. With overdose: severe dizziness, severe drowsiness, cold or clammy skin, mental confusion, seizures or severe restlessness — notify physician.

Warnings: Long-term use may cause physical and psychological dependence and tolerance. Causes birth defects in animals — avoid during first three months of pregnancy. Known to be present in mothers' milk — avoid drug or avoid nursing. Should be used with extreme caution by patients with glaucoma, asthma attacks, epilepsy, impaired kidney or liver function.

Possible Interactions: Sedation may increase when taken with: tranquilizers, antihistamines, antidepressants, sedatives, sleep inducers, alcohol, narcotics and phenothiazines. Serious reactions may occur if MAO inhibitors are taken within 14 days of meperidine hydrochloride.

Mephobarbital
See: Barbiturate Class

Meprobamate

Brand Name: Equanil®

Category Of Drug: Tranquilizer

Intended Effects: To relieve tension and anxiety, to promote sleep.

Side Effects: Drowsiness, incoordinated movements, dizziness, slurred speech, headache, loss of balance, weakness, tingling sensations, difficulty in focusing eyes, elevated mood, overstimulation, nausea, vomiting, diarrhea, pounding heartbeat, skipped heartbeats and other disturbances of heart rhythm, low blood pressure, skin rashes with itching, blood disorders, fluid retention, fever, severe hypersensitive reactions such as chills, restricted breathing and shock.

Warnings: Drug dependence may develop. Sudden withdrawal from the drug after taking it for a period of weeks may cause severe anxiety, tremors, hallucinations or convulsions. Dosage should be reduced gradually after taking the drug for a period of several weeks. Not for children under 6 years of age. Not for people who are allergic to carbromal, carisoprodol, or mebutamate. Should be used with great caution by epileptics, or people with impaired liver or kidney function. Because of possible drowsiness, drive and operate machinery with caution. Causes birth defects in animals — avoid during first three months of pregnancy. Known to be present in mothers' milk — avoid drug or avoid nursing.

Possible Interactions: May change seizure pattern if taken with anticonvulsants. Sedation may increase when taken with: tranquilizers, antihistamines, antidepressants, sedatives, sleep inducers, alcohol and narcotics.

Metaproterenol

Brand Name: Alupent®

Category of Drug: Bronchial-Tube Relaxer (systemic), Decongestant

Intended Effects: To relieve spasms in asthma, bronchitis and emphysema, to reduce tightness in chest.

Side Effects: High blood pressure, irregular or rapid heartbeat, heart disease, glaucoma, fear, anxiety, restlessness, insomnia, tension, convulsions, tremor, loss of balance, weakness, dizziness, flushing, headache, nausea, vomiting, sweating, anorexia, muscle cramps, anginal pain, pallor, difficult or painful urination. With overdose: convulsions, hallucinations, serious breathing problems, fever, chills, vomiting, cold perspiration.

Warnings: Should be taken with caution by those with stroke, angina, high blood pressure, diabetes, overactive thyroid, history of seizures, glaucoma, or prostate over-development. A sharp rise in blood pressure may cause stroke or bleeding.

Possible Interactions: Serious side effects can occur if this drug is taken with or soon after taking another bronchial-tube relaxer or decongestant in pill or liquid form.

Methenamine Mandelate

Brand Name: Mandelamine®

Category Of Drug: Anti-infective

Intended Effects: To treat kidney or urinary tract infections.

Side Effects: Skin rash, stomach irritation, nausea, vomiting. With large doses: bladder irritation, frequent or painful urination.

Warnings: May cause birth defects — avoid or use cautiously during first three months of pregnancy. Not for those with severely impaired liver or kidney function or for people whose urine cannot or should not be acidified.

Possible Interactions: Diuretics, antacids and acetazolamide may decrease its effectiveness. Mandelamine® and sulfonamides may combine to cause dangerous crystal formations in the kidneys — avoid this combination.

Methocarbamol

Brand Name: Robaxin®

Category Of Drug: Muscle Relaxant, Sedative

Intended Effects: To relieve discomfort associated with painful muscle tension.

Side Effects: Lightheadedness, dizziness, drowsiness, nausea, hives, itching, rash, inflammation of the eyelids, nasal congestion, blurred vision, headache, fever.

Warnings: Not for children under the age of 12. Known to be present in mothers' milk — avoid drug or avoid nursing.

Possible Interactions: Sedation may increase when taken with: tranquilizers, antihistamines, antidepressants, sedatives, sleep inducers, alcohol and narcotics. May reduce the effectiveness of pyridostigmine.

Methyclothiazide
See: Thiazide Diuretic Class

Methyldopa

Brand Name: Aldomet®

Category Of Drug: Blood-Pressure Reducer

Intended Effects: To lower blood pressure.

Side Effects: Drowsiness, headache, dizziness, weakness during first few weeks of treatment, tiredness, light-headedness, dry mouth, stuffy nose. Less frequent: skin rash, joint and muscle discomfort, nausea, vomiting, diarrhea, water retention, breast enlargement, impotence, Parkinson-like palsy disorders, inflammation of the pancreas, behavioral changes. Rare: reduction of white blood cell count, liver disorders, hepatitis, bone-marrow depression, fever, nightmares.

Warnings: May cause severe anemia or liver disorders. Not intended for treatment of mild or uncomplicated cases of high blood pressure. May be necessary to adjust dosage during hot weather. Emotional depression should be promptly reported to physician. Known to be present in mothers' milk — avoid drug or avoid nursing.

Possible Interactions: Alcohol can exaggerate the sedative effect and increase ability to lower blood pressure — use with extreme caution. Increases the effects of other blood-pressure reducers, anticlotting drugs, tolbutamide, or lithium. May cause loss of bladder control when taken with phenoxybenzamine. May cause behavior disturbances when taken with haloperidol. Avoid taking with tricyclic antidepressants or MAO inhibitor drugs since this combination may cause elevation of the blood pressure. Amphetamines decrease the effectiveness of this medicine. Thiazide diuretics increase its effects. Interacts with cough, cold or allergy medications.

Methyldopa + Chlorothiazide
See: Methyldopa
See: Thiazide Diuretics

Methyldopa + Hydrochlorothiazide
See: Methyldopa
See: Thiazide Diuretics

Methyldopa + Thiazide Diuretics
See: Methyldopa
See: Thiazide Diuretics

Methylphenidate

Brand Name: Ritalin®

Category Of Drug: Stimulant

Intended Effects: To stabilize behavior in children that are over-active, impulsive, or have emotional problems, short attention spans; to treat mild depression.

Side Effects: Most frequent: nervousness and insomnia. Less frequent: skin rash, hives, fever, reduced appetite, nausea, dizziness, rapid and strong heartbeat, headache, drowsiness, pulse and blood pressure changes, abdominal pain, chest pain. With long use: weight loss. Rare: visual disturbances and loss of scalp hair.

Warnings: Not for children under the age of six. Not for treatment of extreme anxiety, tiredness, agitation, tension, severe depression, or for people with glaucoma. Should be used with caution by people with history of seizures or high blood pressure. Tolerance or drug dependence may develop with long-term use.

Possible Interactions: May reduce the effects of guanethidine. May increase blood pressure if taken with MAO inhibitors. If taken with anticonvulsants, changes in seizure pattern may occur. Increases the effects of anticlotting drugs, phenylbutazone and antidepressants.

Methylprednisolone
See: Adrenocorticoid-Systemic or Topical

Methyprylon

Brand Name: Noludar®

Category Of Drug: Sleeping Aid

Intended Effects: To aid or induce sleep.

Side Effects: Morning drowsiness, dizziness, diarrhea, nausea, vomiting, headache, excitation, skin rash, hallucinations, convulsions, confusion, depression, nightmares, blurred vision, constipation, increased awareness of dreaming.

Warnings: Should be used with caution by people with kidney or liver impairment. Use alcohol with caution. Not recommended for children under the age of 12. Because of possible drowsiness, drive and operate machinery with caution.

Possible Interactions: Sedation may increase when taken with: tranquilizers, antihistamines, antidepressants, sedatives, sleep inducers, alcohol and narcotics.

Metoclopramide

Brand Name: Reglan®

Category Of Drug: Antivomiting, Anti-nausea, Anti-heartburn.

Intended Effects: To relieve symptoms of stomach and intestinal inflammation; to relieve vomiting associated with cancer chemo-therapy. To treat anorexia. To relieve stomach problems associated with diabetes.

Side Effects: Most frequent: restlessness, drowsiness, tiredness, laziness. Less frequent: inability to sleep, headache, dizziness, nausea, bowel disturbances, reflex muscle actions. Rare: depression, involuntary muscle movements.

Warnings: Not for people with stomach or intestinal bleeding or problems, pheochromocytoma (tumors), epilepsy, or people taking drugs to control seizures. Use with caution by people with insulin-controlled diabetes.

Possible Interactions: Narcotics and anticholinergic drugs decrease its effects. Sedation may increase when taken with: tranquilizers, antihistamines, antidepressants, sedatives, sleep inducers, alcohol or narcotics. May decrease absorption of drugs, like digoxin, from the stomach. May increase absorption of drugs, like acetaminophen, tetracycline, levodopa, and ethanol, from the small bowel. Insulin may begin to act and lead to hypoglycemia before food has left the stomach. Because Reglan® affects food digestion, insulin dosage or timing may need to be adjusted.

Metolazone
See: Thiazide Diuretic Class

Metoprolol
See: Beta-Adrenergic Blocking Agent Class

Metronidazole

Brand Name: Flagyl®

Category Of Drug: Antiprotozoa, Antibacterial

Intended Effects: To treat certain protozoa infections, usually in the vagina.

Side Effects: Most frequent: nausea, headache, loss of appetite. Less frequent: vomiting, diarrhea, abdominal cramping, constipation, metallic taste in the mouth, furry tongue, sore throat, low white blood count, changes in heartbeat, seizures, dizziness, vertigo, tingling sensations, incoordination, confusion, irritability, depression, weakness, insomnia, hives, rashes, flushing of the skin, nasal congestion, dryness of mouth, dry vagina or vulva, fever, cystitis, urinary problems, a sense of pelvic pressure, dark urine, decreased sex drive, infection by non-susceptible micro-organisms such as yeast-like fungus.

Warnings: Avoid alcohol completely to avoid severe reaction. Causes tumors in animals — avoid during pregnancy. Known to be present in mothers' milk — avoid drug or avoid nursing. Use with caution in people with decreased liver function, those addicted to alcohol, disease of the blood cells or bone marrow. Consult physician if confusion, muscle jerking, weakness in the extremities, or unsteady walking occur. These symptoms may indicate poisonous reaction.

Possible Interactions: May increase effects of warfarin and other anticlotting drugs. May interact with alcohol to cause cramps, nausea, vomiting, headaches and flushing of the skin. If taken with disulfiram (Antabuse®), severe behavior and emotional problems may develop.

Mexiletine

Brand Name: Mexitil®

Category Of Drug: Heart-Rhythm Regulator

Intended Effects: To regulate heart action, to reduce disturbances of heart rhythm.

Side Effects: Most frequent (1-40%): upset stomach, lightheadedness, tremor, coordination difficulties, nausea, vomiting, heartburn, nervousness, awareness of heartbeat, chest pain, headache, blurred vision, changes in sleep habits, loss of feeling, numbness, weakness, tiredness, ringing in the ears, confusion, rash, water retention, irregular heartbeat, diarrhea, constipation, changes in appetite, stomach pain, speech difficulties, depression, dry mouth, difficult breathing, fever. Less frequent (less than 1%): fainting, hot flashes, high blood pressure, loss of memory, loss of consciousness, difficult urinary, impotence, changes in sex drive, sweating, inflammation of the throat. Rare (reported but unconfirmed): low blood pressure, angina, slow heartbeat, hallucinations, convulsions, seizures, peptic ulcer, bleeding in the stomach, abnormal liver function tests, reduction in the number of white blood cells, altered taste, changes in salivation, hair loss, hiccups, dry skin.

Warnings: Should not be used in people with blocked heart arteries, unless a pacemaker is present. Effectiveness of this drug should be closely monitored by a physician as it can cause worsening of the heart-rhythm. Should be used with caution in people with sinus node dysfunction, abnormal conduction within the veins, low blood pressure, history of seizures, liver disease or congestive heart failure. People with severe liver disease may need reduced doses of mexiletine. Known to be present in mothers' milk — avoid drug or avoid nursing.

Possible Interactions: Phenytoin, rifampin and phenobarbital reduce the effects of mexiletine. Cimetidine has been shown to raise mexiletine levels. Should not be used with drugs or strict diet that alters the pH levels of the urine. Magnesium-aluminum hydroxide reduces the effect of mexiletine. Should be taken with food to reduce stomach irritation.

Mexitil® (*Boehringer Ingelheim*)
  See: Mexiletine

Miconazole

Brand Names: Monistat® 3, Monistat® 7

Category Of Drug: Antifungus

Intended Effects: To treat specific fungus infections in the vagina.

Side Effects: Frequent (6%): itching, burning or irritation. Infrequent (less than 1%): vaginal burning, pelvic cramps, hives, skin rash, headache.

Warnings: Consult physician if irritation or sensitization occurs — it may be necessary to stop this treatment. Since Monistat® is absorbed in small amounts, it should be used with caution during pregnancy. Use this drug for full course of therapy — do not discontinue if symptoms disappear.

Micro-K® (*Robins*)
  See: Potassium Supplement Class

Micronase® (*Upjohn*)
  See: Antidiabetic Class

Micronor® (*Ortho*)
  See: Progestin Class

Midrin® (*Carnrick*)

Category Of Drug: Sedative, Blood-Vessel Narrower

Ingredients: Isometheptene Mucate + Dichloralphenazone + Acetaminophen

Intended Effects: To relieve migraine, vascular and tension headaches.

Side Effects: Dizziness, skin rash.

Warnings: Not for people with glaucoma, severe kidney

disease, high blood pressure, liver disease, or organic heart disease. Should be used with caution by people with heart disease or by people who have had recent heart attacks.

Possible Interactions: May cause severe rise in blood pressure if taken with MAO inhibitors.

Miltown® (*Wallace*)
  See: Meprobamate

Mineral Oil
  See: Laxative-Lubricant Class

Note: No Rx prescription required

Minipress® (*Pfizer*)
  See: Prazosin

Minocin® (*Lederle*)
  See: Tetracycline Class

Minocycline
  See: Tetracycline Class

Modane® (*Adria*)
  See: Laxative-Stimulant Class

Note: Also available as Modane® Bulk (see Laxative- Bulk

Class) or as Modane® Soft (see Laxative- Emollient Class)

Note: No Rx prescription required

Modicon® (*Ortho*)
See: Estrogen + Progestin Class

Moduretic® (*Merck Sharp & Dohme*)
See: Amiloride

Monistat® 3 (*Ortho*)
See: Miconazole

Monistat® 7 (*Ortho*)
See: Miconazole

Monoamine Oxidase (MAO) Inhibitor Class

Generic/Brand Names:
Pargyline /Eutonyl® Filmtabs®
Pargyline + Methyclothiazide /Eutron®
Phenelzine Sulfate /Nardil®
Tranylcypromine Sulfate /Parnate®

Category Of Drug: Antidepressant

Intended Effects: To relieve severe emotional depression.

Side Effects: Most serious: fast, sharp rise in blood pressure, headache, awareness of heartbeat, stiff or sore neck, nausea, vomiting, fever, sweating, cold and clammy skin. Most frequent: insomnia, dizziness, weakness. Less frequent: overstimulation, restlessness, drowsiness, dry mouth, diarrhea, abdominal pain, constipation, loss of appetite, fluid retention, blurred vision, chills, impotence, and change in blood sugar levels in diabetics. Rare: hepatitis and skin rash.

Warnings: Not for people with advanced heart disease, adrenalin-producing tumor, liver disease, high blood pressure, history of frequent or severe headaches, or people over the age of 60. Avoid alcohol and follow diet recommended by physician. MAO inhibitors may suppress pain that would serve as a warning for heart problems. Should be used with caution by people with coronary heart disease, diabetes, schizophrenia, poor kidney function, epilepsy or overactive thyroid. Known to be present in mothers' milk — avoid drug or avoid nursing.

Possible Interactions: Should not be taken in combination with other MAO inhibitors, ephedrine, epinephrine, stimulants, appetite suppressants, diuretics, anesthetics, cheese or excessive quantities of caffeine. Do not take with over-the-counter preparations for colds, hay fever or weight-reduction since serious side effects may occur. Sedation may increase when taken with: tranquilizers, antihistamines, antidepressants, sedatives, sleep inducers, alcohol and narcotics. To avoid serious interaction, do not take MAO inhibitors within 14 days of other prescription drugs.

Motrin® (*Upjohn*)
See: Ibuprofen

Mycolog® (*Squibb*)

Category Of Drug: Anti-inflammatory, Anti-itching, Antibiotic

Ingredients: Nystatin + Neomycin + Gramicidin + Triamcinolone

Intended Effects: To combat superficial bacterial infections or yeast-like infections of the skin, penis and vulva.

Side Effects: Burning, itching, irritation, dryness, blistering, redness, swelling, other kinds of fungus infections, loss of pigmentation, impairment of hearing and kidney function.

Warnings: The possibility of side effects increases dramatically if large areas are treated, since the amount of the drugs that can be absorbed into the body's system is greatly increased. Side effects should be minor if Mycolog® is applied to a small area. Not for virus skin diseases. Not for use in the eye, the external ear in people with perforated eardrums, or for people with impaired circulation. Prolonged use may lead to infections by other organisms.

Mycostatin® Oral (*Squibb*)
See: Nystatin

Mycostatin® Topical (*Squibb*)
See: Nystatin

Mylanta® (*Stuart*)

Category Of Drug: Antacid

Ingredients: Aluminum Hydroxide + Magnesium Hydroxide + Simethicone

Intended Effects: To relieve heartburn, upset stomach and stomach ulcer pain.

Warnings: Use with caution in people with impaired kidney function or kidney disease.

Possible Interactions: Interacts with medicine containing tetracycline — do not use together.

Note: No Rx prescription required

Mysoline® (*Ayerst*)
See: Primidone

Mysteclin-F® (*Squibb*)

Category Of Drug: Antibiotic, Antifungus

Ingredients: Tetracycline + Amphotericin B

Intended Effects: To treat certain bacterial and fungus infections.

Side Effects: Skin rash, hives, exaggerated sunburn, loss of appetite, vomiting, nausea, diarrhea, irritation of tongue or mouth, sore throat, abdominal cramps or pain, additional infections by other organisms not affected by the drug.

Warnings: May cause permanent discoloration of the teeth of unborn children if taken during the last half of pregnancy or by children under 9. Not for people who are allergic to any tetracycline drug. Should be used with caution by people with kidney problems, asthma, hay fever, allergies.

Possible Interactions: Antacids or iron and mineral preparations may decrease the effects of this drug. Thisdrug may increase the effects of anticlotting drugs.

Nadolol
See: Beta-Adrenergic Blocking Agent Class

Naldecon® (*Bristol*)

Category Of Drug: Decongestant, Antihistamine

Ingredients: Phenylpropanolamine + Phenylephrine + Phenyltoloxamine + Chlorpheniramine

Intended Effects: To relieve nasal congestion and congestion in the eustachian tubes leading to the ears; for relief of runny nose.

Side Effects: Rapid or pounding heart, headache, dizziness, nausea, sedation, restlessness, tremor, weakness, pallor, respiratory difficulty, difficulty in urination, insomnia, hallucinations, convulsions, depression, disturbances in heart rhythm, low blood pressure — possibly leading to shock, drowsiness, dry mouth, loss of appetite, vomiting, nervousness, blurred vision, skin rashes.

Warnings: Not for people with severe heart disease, narrow-angle glaucoma, urinary retention, peptic ulcer. Not advised during an asthma attack or in people who are sensitive to amines such as phenylephrine or antihistamines. Should be used cautiously by people with high blood pressure, diabetes, heart disease, increased pressure within the eyeball, low thyroid, or enlargement of the prostate.

Possible Interactions: Sedation may increase when taken with: tranquilizers, antihistamines, antidepressants, sedatives, sleep inducers, alcohol and narcotics. MAO inhibitors may increase the effects of Naldecon® and cause a rise in blood pressure. Beta blockers may increase Naldecon's® effects.

Nalfon® (*Dista*)
  See: Fenoprofen

Nalidixic Acid

Brand Name: NegGram®

Category Of Drug: Anti-infective

Intended Effects: To treat urinary tract infections.

Side Effects: Drowsiness, weakness, headache, dizziness, lightheadedness, visual disturbances, changes in color perception, difficulty in focusing, double vision or overbrightness of light, abdominal discomfort, vomiting, nausea, diarrhea, skin rash, hives, joint pain and swelling, abnormally low white blood cells. Rare (with overdose): convulsions.

Warnings: Not for people with seizures. Should be used with caution by people with liver disease, severe kidney failure or poor blood circulation to the brain. Avoid undue exposure to direct sunlight. Not for infants under 3 months. Drive and use alcohol with caution. Causes birth defects in animals — avoid during first three months of pregnancy.

Possible Interactions: May increase the effects of anti-clotting drugs. May impair alertness, physical coordination and judgment if used with alcohol.

Naprosyn® (*Syntex*)
See: Naproxen

Naproxen

Brand Names: Anaprox®, Naprosyn®

Category Of Drug: Anti-inflammatory, Pain Reliever, Fever Reducer

Intended Effects: To reduce the inflammation and pain of arthritis; to ease menstrual cramps.

Side Effects: Heartburn, nausea, upset stomach, abdominal pain, constipation, sore throat, diarrhea, vomiting, passing of tarry stools, stomach or intestinal bleeding, headache, drowsiness, dizziness, lightheadedness, skin eruptions, sweating, skin rashes, hives, bleeding under the skin, ringing in the ears, visual disturbances, hearing disturbances, fluid retention, pounding heartbeat, shortness of breath, prolonged bleeding time. Rare: thirst, jaundice.

Warnings: Should not be given to people who are sensitive to other anti-inflammatory drugs such as aspirin. Use with extreme caution in people who have had stomach or intestinal problems, or poor kidney function. May increase labor time during delivery. May mask signs of infections. Withdraw gradually to avoid increased side effects. Small quantities are known to be present in mothers' milk — use with extreme caution.

Possible Interactions: Aspirin may decrease the effects of Naproxen. Naproxen may increase the effects of anticlotting drugs, phenytoin or antidiabetic drugs.

Nardil® (*Parke-Davis*)
  See: Monoamine Oxidase Inhibitors

Nasalide® (*Syntex*)
  See: Adrenocorticoid Class - Systemic

Natalins® **RX** (*Mead Johnson*)

Category Of Drug: Vitamin/Mineral Supplement

Ingredients: Vitamin A + Vitamin D + Vitamin E + Vitamin C + Folic Acid + Thiamine + Riboflavin + Niacin + Vitamin B6 + Vitamin B12 + Biotin + Pantothenic Acid + Calcium + Iodine + Magnesium + Copper + Zinc.

Intended Effects: To ensure adequate amounts of vitamins and minerals, to prevent anemia during pregnancy.

Warnings: May mask symptoms of anemia caused by lack of Vitamin B12. Not for children, people with Wilson's disease or iron-storage disease. Because of the calcium, use with caution by people with kidney stones.

Navane® (*Roerig*)
See: Thiothixene

NegGram® (*Winthrop*)
See: Nalidixic Acid

Nembutal® (*Abbott*)
See: Barbiturate Class

Neodecadron® Ophthalmic
(*Merck Sharp & Dohme*)
Category Of Drug: Antibiotic, Anti-infective

Ingredients: Neomycin + Dexamethasone

Intended Effects: To treat certain eye infections.

Side Effects: Rare: increased eye pressure, glaucoma, eye nerve damage, cataracts, delayed healing, herpes simplex activation. With long use: fungus infections.

Warnings: Not to be used by patients with virus or

fungus infections in the eye or cornea, chickenpox or cowpox. Notify physician if infection does not respond promptly. Use with extreme caution in people with glaucoma or herpes simplex. May mask or increase existing infection.

Neosporin® Ointment (*Burroughs Wellcome*)

Category Of Drug: Anti-infective

Ingredients: Neomycin + Polymyxin B + Bacitracin

Intended Effects: To treat certain infections such as infected burns, skin grafts and eczema, to prevent bacterial contamination in burns, skin grafts, incisions.

Side Effects: Itching, rash, swelling, or other signs of irritation. Rare: loss of hearing.

Warnings: Caution should be used when treating extensive burns or other extensive conditions where a great amount of absorption is possible, because of increased chance of hearing loss through absorption. Not for use on the eye or outer ear canal if patient has perforated eardrum. Additional infections may develop, especially with prolonged use. People allergic to kanamycin, paromomycin, or streptomycin may also be allergic to this drug.

Note: No Rx prescription required

Neosporin® Ophthalmic (*Burroughs Wellcome*)

Category Of Drug: Anti-infective

Ingredients: Polymyxin B + Neomycin + Gramicidin

Intended Effects: To treat eye infections caused by certain micro-organisms.

Side Effects: Burning, itching or other allergic reactions.

Warnings: Other infections may develop. Preventing the tip of the applicator from touching the eyelid or surrounding area will help keep the solution sterile. People allergic to kanamycin, paromomycin, streptomycin or gentamicin may also be allergic to this drug.

Nicobid® (*USV*)
See: Nicotinic Acid

Nicorette® (*Merrell Dow*)

Category Of Drug: Smoking Deterrent

Ingredient: Nicotine Resin Complex

Intended Effects: To provide non-addictive nicotine as a temporary aid to the cigarette smoker who is trying to quit.

Side Effects: Caused through excessive or hard chewing of the gum: traumatic injury to the teeth or mucous membrane of the mouth, jaw, mouth or throat soreness, belching (from swallowing air). Overall effects: excess saliva, dizziness, lightheadedness, upset stomach, indigestion, nausea, vomiting, hiccups, rapid heartbeat, laxative effect, constipation, gas pains, dry mouth, hoarseness, flushing, sneezing, coughing, excessive feeling of happiness, inability to sleep, heart problems.

Warnings: Not for use by non-smokers, people with serious heart problems, chest pains, active temporomandibular joint disease (TMJ), or recovering from heart attacks. Use with caution by people with over-active thyroid, minor heart or circulation problems, diabetes, throat infections, dental problems, high blood pressure or history of ulcers. May cause severe birth defects — avoid during pregnancy. Should be avoided by women of childbearing potential if not using effective contraception. Known to be present in mothers' milk — avoid drug or avoid nursing.

The nicotine is absorbed through the lining of the mouth. Chew each piece very slowly until you taste the gum, then stop. After the taste is gone, chew again. Most of the listed side effects can be reduced by chewing very slowly. Each piece should last at least 30 minutes. Do not exceed 30 pieces of gum per day.

Possible Interactions: Decreases effects of phenacetin, caffeine, theophylline, imipramine, furosemide and pentazocine. Causes increased blood pressure when taken with propranolol. Increases circulating cortisol and catecholamines — therapy with adrenergic agonists or blockers (beta blockers) may need to be adjusted. When intake of nicotine stops, all these interactions may be reversed and dosages adjusted.

Nicotinic Acid

Brand Name: Nicobid®

Category Of Drug: Blood-Vessel Enlarger, Vitamin Supplement

Intended Effects: To increase blood circulation, to reduce cholesterol levels, to treat nicotinic acid deficiency.

Side Effects: Flushing and feeling of warmth, upset stomach, dry skin, low blood pressure, headache, itching, tingling, rash, nausea, vomiting, abdominal pain, diarrhea. Rare: jaundice and thickening of the skin.

Warnings: Not for people with impaired liver function, peptic ulcer, glaucoma, diabetes, gout, chronic diarrhea, or any bleeding disorder. Causes birth defects in animals — avoid during first three months of pregnancy. Use alcohol with caution.

Possible Interactions: Nicotine, in tobacco, may reduce its effectiveness. May decrease the effects of antidiabetic drugs by raising the level of blood sugar. May increase the effects of some blood-pressure reducers and cause extreme lowering of blood pressure.

Nitrate Class

Generic / Brand Names:
  Isosorbide Dinitrate / Isordil®, Sorbitrate®
  Pentaerythritol Tetranitrate / Peritrate®, Peritrate® SA

Category Of Drug: Blood-Vessel Enlarger

Intended Effects: For the treatment of acute anginal attacks and for the prevention of such attacks in patients suffering from heart disease causing coronary insufficiency. It is not intended to stop an attack once it begins, but is widely regarded as useful in the prevention of angina pectoris.

Side Effects: Reddening or flushing of the skin, headache, dizziness, weakness, nausea, vomiting, restlessness, pallor, perspiration, collapse, and rashes.

Warnings: Tolerance to nitrate drugs may develop and withdrawal may produce anginal pain. People who are allergic to aspirin may also be allergic to some nitrates.

Possible Interactions: Can antagonize the action of norepinephrine, acetylcholine, or histamine. Blood-pressure reducers or alcohol may cause a severe drop in blood pressure when taken with nitrates. Effects can be decreased or altered when taken with many over-the-counter medications for colds and allergies — use with caution.

Nitro-Bid® (*Marion*)
  See: Nitroglycerin-Systemic

Nitrodisc® (*Searle*)
  See: Nitroglycerin-Topical

Nitro-Dur® (*Key*)
  See: Nitroglycerin -Topical

Nitrofurantoin Macrocrystals

Brand Name: Macrodantin®

Category Of Drug: Anti-infective

Intended Effects: To treat urinary tract infections.

Side Effects: Most frequent: nausea, vomiting and loss of appetite. Less frequent: abdominal pain, diarrhea, brown discoloration of the urine (harmless). Infrequent: fever, chills, cough, chest pain, throat and lung congestion, skin rashes, itching, asthma attacks, jaundice, pain in the joints, anemia and other blood disorders, headache, dizziness, rapid eye movements, drowsiness, loss of hair and fungus infections. Rare: hepatitis.

Warnings: Use with caution in cases with asthma, since increased lung congestion can be dangerous; lung reactions may come about gradually. Should not be used in cases of impaired kidney function. Should not use in later stages of pregnancy near delivery or in infants within one month of birth because of the possibility of anemia.

Nitroglycerin - Systemic

Brand Names: Aerosol Spray — Nitrolingual®
Tablets — Nitrostat®, Nitro-Bid®

Category Of Drug: Blood-Vessel Enlarger

Intended Effects: To open arteries by relaxing smooth muscles, and provide increased circulation into the heart in cases of coronary insufficiency, to quickly reduce the pain (angina pectoris) associated with coronary insufficiency caused by heart disease.

Side Effects: Headache, reddening or flushing of the skin, dizziness, weakness, rashes, nausea, vomiting, blurred vision, dry mouth.

Warnings: Tolerance may develop and reduce its

effectiveness. Should be used with caution by people with glaucoma, severe anemia or early signs of heart attack. Tablets loose potency in 3 months after they are opened. Refrigerate unused portions to keep them potent.

Possible Interactions: Cross-tolerance develops between nitroglycerin and other organic nitrites. When taken with alcohol or blood pressure reducers may cause a severe drop in blood pressure.

Nitroglycerin-Topical

Brand Names: Ointment — Nitrol®
Skin pad — Nitrodisc®, Nitro-Dur®, Transderm-Nitro®

Category Of Drug: Blood-Vessel Enlarger

Intended Effects: To open arteries by relaxing smooth muscles, and provide increased circulation into the heart in cases of coronary insufficiency, to quickly reduce the pain (angina pectoris) associated with coronary insufficiency caused by heart disease.

Side Effects: Headache, reddening or flushing of the skin, dizziness, weakness, rashes, nausea, vomiting, blurred vision, dry mouth.

Warnings: Follow directions on dose-measuring application papers which are supplied with the medicine. For external use only. The ointment form of this medicine is not for relief of an acute angina attack because of the slow rate of action. Tolerance may develop and reduce its effects. Should be used with caution by people with glaucoma, severe anemia or heart malfunctions.

Possible Interactions: Cross-tolerance develops between nitroglycerin and other organic nitrites. When taken with alcohol or blood pressure reducers may cause a severe drop in blood pressure.

Nitrol® (*Rorer*)
  See: Nitroglycerin-Topical

Nitrolingual® (*Rorer*)
  See: Nitroglycerin-Systemic

Nitrostat® (*Parke-Davis*)
  See: Nitroglycerin-Systemic

Noctec® (*Squibb*)
  See: Chloral Hydrate

Nolamine® (*Carnrick*)

Category Of Drug: Decongestant, Antihistamine

Ingredients: Chlorpheniramine + Phenindamine Tartrate + Phenylpropanolamine

Intended Effects: To relieve nasal congestion caused by allergies, the common cold, or sinus inflammation.

Side Effects: Drowsiness, tremors, dizziness, nervousness, insomnia.

Warnings: Due to possible drowsiness, drive and operate machinery with caution. Should be used with caution by people with high blood pressure, diabetes, heart disease or overactive thyroid.

Possible Interactions: Sedation may increase when taken with: tranquilizers, antihistamines, antidepressants, sedatives, sleep inducers, alcohol and narcotics. May decrease the effects of anticlotting drugs. Do NOT use with MAO inhibitors.

Noludar® (*Roche*)
See: Methyprylon

Nordette® (*Wyeth*)
See: Estrogen + Progestin Class

Norethindrone
See: Progestin Class

Norethindrone + Ethinyl Estradiol
See: Estrogen + Progestin Class

Norethindrone + Mestranol
See: Estrogen + Progestin Class

Norethynodrel + Mestranol
See: Estrogen + Progestin Class

Norgesic® (*Riker*)

Category Of Drug: Muscle Relaxant, Pain Reliever

Ingredients: Orphenadrine + Aspirin + Caffeine

Intended Effects: To relax muscles and relieve pain associated with muscle injuries.

Side Effects: Rapid or pounding heartbeat, retention of urine, dry mouth, blurred vision, wide pupils, increased pressure within the eyeball, weakness, nausea, vomiting, headache, dizziness, constipation, drowsiness, hives, mental confusion, excitation, hallucinations, anemia, bleeding, lightheadedness, blacking out.

Warnings: Not for patients with glaucoma, stomach obstruction, enlarged prostate, obstructions at the bladder neck, or those with myasthenia gravis. Should be used with extreme caution by people with peptic ulcers and bleeding problems. Not recommended for children under the age of 12. Drive and operate machinery with caution.

Possible Interactions: Confusion, anxiety and tremors may result from combination of propoxyphene and Norgesic®. Many over-the-counter medicines for colds, coughs, and allergies may interact unfavorably with this drug. Sedation may increase when taken with: tranquilizers, antihistamines, antidepressants, sedatives, sleep inducers, alcohol and narcotics. May increase the action of anticlotting drugs.

Norgesic® Forte
See: Norgesic®

Note: FORTE means" extra strength".

Norgestrel
See: Progestin Class

Norgestrel + Ethinyl Estradiol
See: Estrogen + Progestin Class

Norinyl® (*Syntex*)
See: Estrogen + Progestin Class

Norlestrin® (*Parke-Davis*)
See: Estrogen + Progestin Class

Norlestrin® FE (*Parke-Davis*)
See: Estrogen + Progestin Class

Note: Same as Norlestrin®, plus brown tablets which are iron supplements.

Norlutate® (*Parke-Davis*)
See: Progestin Class

Normodyne® (*Schering*)
See: Labetalol

Norpace® (*Searle*)
See: Disopyramide

Norpramin® (*Merrell Dow*)
See: Tricyclic Antidepressant Class

Novafed® (*Merrell Dow*)
See: Pseudoephedrine

Novafed® A (*Merrell Dow*)
See: Pseudoephedrine
See: Antihistamine Class

Novahistine® Expectorant (*Merrell Dow*)

Category Of Drug: Anticough, Decongestant, Phlegm Loosener

Ingredients: Codeine + Phenylpropanolamine + Guaifenesin + Alcohol

Intended Effects: To loosen phlegm associated with cough and respiratory congestion, to relieve coughing, to reduce nasal and eustachian tube (ear) congestion.

Side Effects: Nausea, vomiting, constipation, dizziness, sedation, pounding heartbeat, itching, difficult breathing. Rare: high blood pressure.

Warnings: Should be used with caution by people with high blood pressure, heart disease, emphysema, asthma, diabetes, thyroid disease, increased pressure within the eye, enlarged prostate. Not for use by people with severe high blood pressure, severe coronary artery disease, people taking MAO inhibitors, or nursing mothers.

Possible Interactions: May decrease the effects of blood-pressure reducers. Beta blockers and MAO inhibitors increase its effects. Sedation may increase when taken with: tranquilizers, antihistamines, antidepressants, sedatives, sleep inducers, alcohol and narcotics.

Note: No Rx prescription required

Nylidrin

Brand Name: Arlidin®

Category Of Drug: Blood-Vessel Enlarger

Intended Effects: To relieve dizziness or loss of balance associated with poor circulation of blood in the inner ear, relief of symptoms associated with poor circulation of blood in the limbs.

Side Effects: Nervousness, weakness, dizziness, tremor, nausea, vomiting, rapid heartbeat, acid indigestion, continuing weakness or tiredness, irregular heartbeat.

Warnings: Use alcohol with caution until its effects with this drug have been determined. Avoid after recent heart attack, stroke, or peptic ulcer. Use with caution by those with glaucoma, poor brain circulation, stroke,
   coronary heart disease, heart rhythm disorders or overactive thyroid. Use with caution while driving.

Possible Interactions: Smoking should be avoided since nicotine is frequently a major contributing factor to the problem which is being treated and can reduce drug's effectiveness. Cold environments may reduce effectiveness. Nylidrin can increase the effects of thiazide diuretics. Metoprolol, propranolol, timolol and other beta adrenergic blocking agents may decrease the effects of Nylidrin .

Nystatin - Oral

Brand Name: Mycostatin®-Oral

Category Of Drug: Antifungus, Antibiotic

Intended Effects: To treat certain yeast-like fungus infections of the mouth or intestines.

Side Effects: With large doses: diarrhea, stomach pain, nausea and vomiting.

Warnings: May cause allergic-reactions in people who are allergic to aspirin. The oral suspension (syrup) for treatment of mouth and throat infections should be kept in the mouth for as long as possible before swallowing. Use this drug for full course of treatment, even if symptoms have disappeared.

Nystatin - Topical

Brand Name: Mycostatin®-Topical

Category Of Drug: Antifungus, Antibiotic

Intended Effects: To treat certain fungus infections.

Side Effects: Irritation and itching where applied.

Warnings: Use this drug for full course of treatment, even if symptoms have disappeared.

Ogen® (*Abbott*)
See: Estrogen Class-Systemic
See: Estrogen Class-Vaginal

Omnipen® (*Wyeth*)
See: Penicillin Class

Optimine® (*Schering*)
See: Antihistamine Class

Organidin® (*Wallace*)

Category Of Drug: Phlegm Loosener

Ingredients: Iodinated Glycerol

Intended Effects: To ease bronchitis, bronchial asthma, emphysema, cystic fibrosis and chronic sinus inflammation by loosening and thinning mucus and respiratory tract fluid.

Side Effects: Stomach irritation, rash, allergic reactions, acne, enlarged thyroid gland, enlarged salivary glands.

Warnings: Causes birth defects in animals — avoid during pregnancy. Known to be present in mothers' milk — avoid drug or avoid nursing. Use with great caution or avoid use by people with history of thyroid disease. May increase the possibility of goiters in children with cystic fibrosis.

Possible Interactions: This drug may increase the effects of lithium and anti-thyroid drugs.

Orinase® (*Upjohn*)
  See: Antidiabetic Class

Ornade® (*Smith Kline & French*)
  See: Phenylpropanolamine
  See: Antihistamine Class

Note: Rx prescription required only for Spansule® Capsules dosage

---

Ortho-Novum® (*Ortho*)
  See: Estrogen + Progestin Class

Orudis® (*Wyeth Laboratories*)

See: Ketoprofen

Os-Cal® (*Marion*)

Category Of Drug: Vitamin/Mineral Supplement

Ingredients: Calcium + Vitamin D

Intended Effects: To treat calcium deficiency.

Side Effects: With overdose: weakness, fatigue, "unwell" feeling, dry mouth, muscle aches, headache, metallic taste in the mouth. With prolonged overdose: kidney stones, irregular heartbeat, reduced mental abilities, damage to the kidneys, heart, blood vessels and other organs.

Warnings: Calcium requirements should be determined by a physician to avoid the dangerous condition of calcium excess.

Note: No Rx prescription required

Ovcon® (*Mead Johnson*)
See: Estrogen + Progestin Class

Ovral® (*Wyeth*)
See: Estrogen + Progestin Class

Ovrette® (*Wyeth*)
See: Progestin Class

Ovulen® (*Searle*)
See: Estrogen + Progestin Class

Oxazepam
See: Benzodiazepine Class

Oxtriphylline
See: Xanthine Class

Oxybutynin

Brand Name: Ditropan®

Category Of Drug: Antispasmodic

Intended Effects: To help promote bladder control.

Side Effects: Dry mouth, decreased sweating, urinary hesitance and retention, blurred vision, pupil dilation, increased pressure within the eye, drowsiness, dizziness, weakness, insomnia, nausea, vomiting, constipation, bloated feeling, suppression of milk production, impotence, skin rash, rapid heartbeat.

Warnings: Should be used with caution by the elderly, by people with kidney or liver disease, ulcerative colitis or hiatal hernia. This drug may aggravate symptoms of coronary heart disease, congestive heart failure, rapid heartbeat, high blood pressure, prostate problems, overactive thyroid, irregular heartbeat. Caution required while driving or operating machinery due to drowsiness. Not for children under the age of five. In hot weather, heat prostration is possible because of decreased sweating. Should be used with caution by people with iliostomy or colostomy. Not for people with glaucoma, gastrointestinal tract obstruction, severe colitis or myasthenia gravis.

Oxycodone

Category Of Drug: Pain Reliever, Narcotic

Intended Effects: To relieve mild to moderately severe pain, to control coughing.

Side Effects: Most frequent: drowsiness, constipation, unsteady walking, lightheadedness, dizziness, sedation, nausea and vomiting. Less frequent: euphoria, constipation, itching.

Warnings: Should be used with caution in people with poor kidney or liver function, enlarged prostate. Addison's disease, underactive thyroid, head injury or acute abdominal conditions. Not for use by children. Drug dependence may develop. Because of possible drowsiness, drive and operate machinery with caution.

Possible Interactions: Sedation may increase when taken with: tranquilizers, pain relievers, antihistamines, antidepressants, sedatives, sleep inducers, alcohol and narcotics. Oxycodone and phenytoin may combine to cause reduced brain functions. Cyproheptadine or methysergide may decrease its effectiveness.

Panmycin® (*Upjohn*)
See: Tetracycline Class

Papaverine

Brand Name: Pavabid®

Category Of Drug: Blood-Vessel Enlarger

Intended Effects: To relieve blockage or restrictions in the flow of blood in the arteries, to relieve heart spasms, toincrease blood flow, to regulate heartbeat.

Side Effects: Nausea, stomach distress, loss of appetite, constipation, drowsiness, lightheadedness, sweating, headache, diarrhea, skin rash, itching, indigestion, dryness of mouth and throat.

Warnings: Use with caution in cases with glaucoma. May affect liver function. May cause blood disorders including jaundice.

Possible Interactions: Nicotine, in tobacco, can reduce its effectiveness. Sedation may increase when taken with: tranquilizers, antihistamines, sleep inducers, antidepressants, sedatives, alcohol and narcotics.

Parafon Forte® (*McNeil*)

Category Of Drug: Muscle Relaxant, Pain Reliever

Ingredients: Chlorzoxazone + Acetaminophen

Intended Effects: To relax muscle spasms, to provide relief from muscle pain, stiffness, and limitation of motion.

Side Effects: Side effects are rare but the following may occur: drowsiness, dizziness, lightheadedness, uneasiness, over-stimulation, rashes, retention of fluids, shock, bleeding in the stomach or intestines. Liver damage is possible but not confirmed.

Warnings: Should be used with caution by people with impaired liver function or history of liver disease. Overdose may cause liver damage. Known to be present in mothers' milk — avoid drug or avoid nursing.

Possible Interactions: Sedation may increase when taken with: tranquilizers, antihistamines, antidepressants, sedatives, sleep inducers, alcohol and narcotics.

Paregoric

Category Of Drug: Antidiarrhea, Narcotic

Intended Effects: To relieve diarrhea and intestinal cramps, to relieve moderate pain.

Side Effects: Constipation, lightheadedness, sweating, drowsiness, blurred vision, dry mouth, difficult urination, flushing or dryness of skin, hives, itching, skin rash, dizziness, unsteadiness.

Warnings: Not for people with glaucoma, liver or kidney disease, or for people who may be allergic to any opium derivative. The young and the elderly may be more sensitive to its sedative effects. Known to be present in mothers' milk — avoid drug or avoid nursing. Drug dependence may develop with large doses.

Possible Interactions: Sedation may increase when taken with: tranquilizers, antihistamines, sleep inducers, antidepressants, sedatives, alcohol and narcotics.

Pargyline HCl
See: Monoamine Oxidase Inhibitor Class

Parnate® (*Smith Kline & French*)
See: Monoamine Oxidase Inhibitor Class

Pathibamate® (*Lederle*)

Category Of Drug: Antispasm, Tranquilizer

Ingredients: Tridihexethyl Chloride + Meprobamate

Intended Effects: To aid in the treatment of peptic ulcer and irritable bowel syndrome, especially when accompanied by tension or anxiety.

Side Effects: Blurred vision, drowsiness, urinary hesitancy and retention, rapid heartbeat, loss of taste, headaches, nervousness, dizziness, insomnia, nausea, vomiting, suppression of milk production, constipation, bloated feeling, decreased sweating. In the elderly: mental confusion or excitement. Rare: may cause seizures in epileptic patients.

Warnings: Not for those who are unable to empty the bladder completely, or those with severe ulcerative colitis, narrow-angle glaucoma or myasthenia gravis. Drive and operate machinery with caution due to possible blurred visionor drowsiness. Should be used with caution by people with impaired kidney or liver function, coronary heart disease, overactive thyroid, congestive heart failure, high blood pressure, non-obstructing enlarged prostate, hiatus hernia, history of peptic ulcers. Possibility of heat stroke in hot weather exists due to decreased sweating. Not for children under 12. Drug dependence may develop. Discontinue gradually.

Possible Interactions: Sedation may increase when taken with: tranquilizers, antihistamines, sleep inducers, antidepressants, sedatives, alcohol and narcotics.

Pavabid® (*Marion*)
See: Papaverine

PBZ® (*Geigy*)
See: Antihistamine Class

Pediamycin® (*Ross*)
See: Erythromycin Class

Pediazole® (*Ross*)
See: Erythromycin Class
See: Sulfonamide Class - Systemic

Penicillin Class

Generic / Brand Names:
  Amoxicillin/Amoxil®, Augmentin®, Polymox®,
Trimox®, Wymox®
  Ampicillin/Amcill®,Omnipen®,Principen®, Totacillin®
  Bacampicillin/Spectrobid®
  Carbenicillin/Geocillin®
  Cloxacillin Sodium/Tegopen
  Cyclacillin/Cyclapen-W®
  Dicloxacillin
  Penicillin G Potassium/Pentids®
  Penicillin V/Ledercillin® VK, Pen-Vee-K®, Robicillin®
VK, V-Cillin K®
  Penicillin VK-Potassium/Beepen® VK, Pfizerpen® VK

Category Of Drug: Antibiotic

Intended Effects: To combat infections caused by certain organisms.

Side Effects: Nausea, vomiting, diarrhea, black tongue, skin rashes, chills, fever, retention of fluid, pain in the joints, swelling of the larynx, prostration, fever, unusual bruising or bleeding, anemia or other blood disorders. Rare: anaphylactic shock.

Warnings: Should not be taken by anyone with a history of sensitivity to penicillin or cephalosporin antibiotics. Should be taken with caution by people who have a history of other allergic reactions. Liquid forms of penicillin should not be taken if medicine is older than 7 days (room temperature) or 14 days (refrigerated). Fungus infections may develop after use. Animal studies show increase in birth defects when taken during pregnancy, but human studies show no increase in birth defects. May be present in mothers' milk — avoid drug or avoid nursing.

Possible Interactions: Other antibiotics may decrease the effectiveness of penicillins or react unfavorably with them.

Penicillin G
See: Penicillin Class

Penicillin V
See: Penicillin Class

Penicillin VK
See: Penicillin Class

Pentaerythritol Tetranitrate
See: Nitrate Class

Pentazocine

Brand Name: Talwin®

Category Of Drug: Pain Reliever

Intended Effects: To relieve moderate to severe pain.

Side Effects: Most frequent: nausea, vomiting, dizziness, lightheadedness, sedation, euphoria, headache, sweating. Infrequent: constipation, weakness, disturbed dreams, insomnia, blackouts, blurred vision, focusing difficulty, hallucinations, rash, low blood pressure, rapid heartbeat. Rare:

abdominal pain, loss of appetite, diarrhea, tremor, irritability, excitement, ringing in the ears, chills, swelling of the face, low white blood cell count and other blood disorders, slowed breathing rate, urinary retention, tingling sensations, destruction of skin.

Warnings: Drug dependence may develop. Abrupt discontinuation may cause withdrawal symptoms. Should not be used in cases of head injury or pressure in the skull. Should be used cautiously by people who have respiratory problems, impaired kidney or liver function, history of heart attack, seizures or bronchial asthma. Not recommended for children under 12. Due to possible drowsiness, drive or operate machinery with caution.

Possible Interactions: Reduces the effectiveness of narcotics and may cause withdrawal symptoms from people who have been taking large doses of narcotics. Sedation may increase when taken with: tranquilizers, antihistamines, antidepressants, sedatives, sleep inducers and alcohol.

Pentids® (*Squibb*)
See: Penicillin Class

Pentobarbital
See: Barbiturate Class

Pentoxifylline

Brand Name: Trental®

Category Of Drug: Anti-cramping, Anti-hemorrhaging

Intended Effects: To treat leg cramps caused by constricted arteries.

Side Effects: Nausea, dizziness, belching, bloating, indigestion, headache, blurred vision, insomnia, drowsiness, nervousness, vomiting, diarrhea, stomach discomfort, chest pain, flushing, awareness of heartbeat, water retention, low blood pressure, loss of appetite, inflammation of the gall bladder, constipation, dry mouth, thirstiness, anxiety, confusion, flu-like symptoms, stuffy nose, tremors, brittle fingernails, itchiness, rash, earache, bad taste, sore throat, swollen neck glands, weight change.

Warnings: Should not be used by people who are allergic to caffeine, theophylline or theobromine. Should be used with caution in people taking blood-pressure reducers. Safety in children has not been established. Should be taken with meals.

Possible Interactions: None known.

Pen-Vee® K (*Wyeth*)
See: Penicillin Class

Percocet®-5 (*Du Pont*)
See: Oxycodone
See: Acetaminophen

Percodan® (*Du Pont*)
See: Oxycodone
See: Salicylate Class

Periactin® (*Merck Sharp & Dohme*)
See: Antihistamine Class

Peritrate® (*Parke-Davis*)
See: NitrateClass

Perphenazine
See: Phenothiazine Class

Persantine® (*Boehringer Ingelheim*)
See:Dipyridamole

Pfizerpen VK® (*Pfipharmecs*)
See: Penicillin Class

Phenaphen® (*Robins*)
See: Acetaminophen

Note: No Rx prescription required

Phenaphen® + Codeine (*Robins*)
See: Acetaminophen
See: Codeine

Phenazopyridine

Brand Names: Pyridium®

Category Of Drug: Pain Reliever

Intended Effects: To relieve pain, burning and other dis-
comforts caused by irritation of the lower urinary tract due to
infection as in cystitis, injury, surgery, or catheterization.

Side Effects: Orange-red discoloration of urine is typical
and not a problem. Skin rash, indigestion, abdominal
cramps, dizziness, headache. Rare (usually with overdose):
blood disorders, kidney damage, liver damage.

Warnings: Not for patients with poor kidney function or
hepatitis. This drug is intended only to relieve symptoms.
Additional medication is required to cure infections. Known
to be present in mothers' milk — avoid drug or avoid nursing. May interfere with milk production. Urine color may
permanently stain clothing.

Phenelzine
See: Monoamine Oxidase Inhibitor Class

Phenergan® (*Wyeth*)
See: Promethazine

Phenergan® Expectorant (*Wyeth*)

Category Of Drug: Antihistamine, Phlegm Loosener

Ingredients: Promethazine + Ipecac + Potassium
Guaiacolsulfonate + Citric Acid + Sodium Citrate

Intended Effects: To relieve congestion due to colds, minor upper respiratory infections, pollen hay fever, and dust sensitivity, to loosen phlegm.

Side Effects: Drowsiness, blurred vision, dizziness, dryness of mouth, nose and throat, nausea, vomiting, ringing in the ears, skin rash, upset stomach, unusual excitement, nervousness, nightmares. Especially in children: restlessness, irritability, decreased alertness. Rare: low white blood cell count and other blood disorders, increases or decreases in blood pressure, light sensitivity.

Warnings: Should be discontinued one to two weeks before delivery to avoid possible harm to the infant. Should be used with caution by those with acute asthma, narrow-angle glaucoma, jaundice, prostate enlargement, history of peptic ulcer, epilepsy, impaired liver function, bone marrow depression, heart disease, children with high fever who may have Reye's syndrome. Not recommended for children under the age of 3 months.

Possible Interactions: May lower the convulsion threshold of anticonvulsants and increase severity of convulsions. Effects of atropine and related compounds may be increased when used with this drug. Any over-the-counter drugs for allergies or colds may interact with this drug. Sedation may increase when taken with: tranquilizers, antihistamines, antidepressants, sedatives, sleep inducers, alcohol and narcotics.

Phenergan® Expectorant + Codeine *(Wyeth)*

Category Of Drug: Antihistamine, Phlegm Loosener, Anticough

Ingredients: Promethazine + Ipecac + Potassium Guaiacolsulfonate + Citric Acid + Sodium Citrate + Codeine

Intended Effects: To reduce coughing in addition to the other activity of Phenergan® Expectorant.

  See: Phenergan® Expectorant
  See: Codeine

Phenergan® Pediatric Expectorant (*Wyeth*)

Category Of Drug: Antihistamine, Phlegm Loosener, Anticough

Ingredients: Promethazine + Ipecac + Potassium Guaiacolsulfonate + Citric Acid + Sodium Citrate + Dextromethorphan

Intended Effects: This combination Phenergan® preparation is marketed as being suitable for children.

Side Effects: **See:** Phenergan® Expectorant.

Warnings: Not recommended for children under the age of three months. Should be used with caution by children with respiratory disorders or high fever who may have Reye's syndrome. **See:** Phenergan® Expectorant.

Possible Interactions: Reacts unfavorably with MAO inhibitor antidepressants. **See:** Phenergan® Expectorant.

Phenergan® Suppositories (*Wyeth*)

Category Of Drug: Antihistamine, Antivomiting, Sedative

Ingredients: Promethazine + Ascorbyl Palmitate + Silicon Dioxide + White Wax + Cocoa Butter

Intended Effects: In addition to other effects: to stop vomiting when orally administered drugs might be vomitted.

See: Promethazine

Phenergan® VC Expectorant (*Wyeth*)

Category Of Drug: Antihistamine, Expectorant, Bronchial Tube Relaxer

Ingredients: Promethazine + Ipecac + Potassium Guaiacolsulfonate + Citric Acid + Sodium Citrate + Phenylephrine

Intended Effects: To reduce chest tightness plus the other intended effects of Phenergan® Expectorant.

See: Phenergan® Expectorant.

Phenergan® VC Expectorant + Codeine
(*Wyeth*)

Category Of Drug: Antihistamine, Expectorant, Bronchial Tube Relaxer, Anticough.

See: Phenergan® VC Expectorant
See: Codeine

Phenmetrazine

See: Appetite Suppressant Class

Phenobarbital
See: Barbiturate Class

Phenolphthalein
See: Laxatives-Stimulant Class

Phenothiazines

Generic / Brand Names:
Chlorpromazine/Thorazine®
Fluphenazine/Prolixin®
Perphenazine/Trilafon®
Perphenazine + Amitriptyline/Triavil®
Prochlorperazine/Compazine®
Thioridazine/Mellaril®
Trifluoperazine/Stelazine®

Category Of Drug: Tranquilizer

Intended Effects: To treat schizophrenia, manic- depressive illness, and psychotic manifestations of mental illness. To control nausea and vomiting, to relieve apprehension before surgery, to help in the treatment of tetanus, to relieve severe hiccups, to control hyperactivity and other behavior disorders in children.

Side Effects: Rolling motions of the tongue and other involuntary movements, especially in elderly patients who have been taking phenothiazines for a long time. (**Note:**

Recent studies indicate that large doses of B vitamins taken with phenothiazines can greatly reduce the danger of brain damage causing loss of muscle control). Drowsiness, jaundice, blood disorders, low blood pressure, rashes including light-sensitive rashes, signs of feminization including milk flow and breast enlargement, skipped menstrual periods, dry mouth, nasal congestion, constipation, retention of urine, increased appetite and weight, fluid retention, reduction in the coughing reflex.

Warnings: Avoid use in children and adolescents with high fever who may have Reye's syndrome. Should be used with caution in people who have a history of respiratory disorders such as asthma, emphysema, and respiratory infections. Should be used cautiously in people who have heart, blood vessel or liver disease. Do not stop abruptly. Known to be present in mothers' milk — avoid drug or avoid nursing.

Possible Interactions: Sedation may increase when taken with: tranquilizers, sleep inducers, antihistamines, antidepressants, sedatives, alcohol and narcotics. Interacts with many over-the-counter medicines for colds, allergies and coughs. Smoking reduces blood plasma concentrations dramatically. Dosage adjustments may be necessary.

Phentermine

See: Appetite Suppressant Class

Phenylbutazone Class

Generic/Brand Name:
Phenylbutazone/Butazolidin®

Category Of Drug: Anti-inflammatory, Fever Reducer, Pain Reliever, Anti-arthritic

Intended Effects: To relieve symptoms of gouty arthritis, rheumatoid arthritis, or certain joint diseases (degenerative arthritis, bursitis).

Side Effects: Nausea, indigestion, heartburn, abdominal discomfort, anemia, skin rash, fluid retention, kidney problems, headache, drowsiness, vomiting, diarrhea. Rare: high fever, severe sore throat, unusual bleeding or bruising, sudden weight gain, enlarged salivary glands, kidney damage, hepatitis, high blood pressure.

Warnings: Should be taken with milk or at mealtimes. Should not be taken by children 14 or younger, patients with serious heart problems, inflammation of the pancreas, serious liver or kidney problems, or symptoms of stomach or intestinal ulcers. Patients experiencing visual disturbances should report them immediately and have an eye exam. Should be used with care in the elderly, and not at all in the senile. May provoke asthma attacks. May interfere with thyroid tests. Caution should be used if driving or operating machinery. Causes birth defects in animals — avoid during first three months of pregnancy. Known to be present in mothers' milk — avoid drug or avoid nursing.

Possible Interactions: Salt intake may need to be restricted. Alcohol may increase its drowsiness effects. Aspirin, barbiturates or antidepressants may reduce its effectiveness. May decrease the action of digitalis medicines antihistamines, and oral contraceptives. May increase the effects of anticlotting drugs, insulin, lithium, penicillins, sulfonamides and antidiabetic drugs.

Phenylpropanolamine

Category Of Drug: Decongestant, Appetite Suppressant, Antihistamine

Intended Effects: To relieve congestion of sinuses, nose and throat associated with infections and allergies; to suppress appetite.

Side Effects: Insomnia, unusually fast, irregular or pounding heartbeat, nervousness, headache, dizziness, nausea, restlessness, blood pressure increase, vomiting.

Warnings: Contained in many over-the-counter drugs for colds, allergies and coughs — combinations of these drugs may produce unfavorable effects. Do not exceed recommended dose — large doses may cause rise in blood pressure. People sensitive to epinephrine, ephedrine, terbutaline and amphetamines may also be sensitive to this drug. Should be used with caution by people with high blood pressure, overactive thyroid, diabetes or heart disease.

Possible Interactions: May increase the effects of epinephrine. May decrease the effects of blood-pressure reducers. If taken with digitalis preparations, serious disturbances of heart rhythm may result. If taken with guanethidine, effectiveness of both drugs may be reduced. If taken with ergot preparations, serious rise in blood pressure may result. Tricyclic antidepressants may interact to cause excess stimulation of the heart and blood pressure. Do not take within 14 days of MAO inhibitors to avoid dangerous rise in blood pressure.

Note: This drug is available in combination form

without prescription in many products for coughs, allergies and colds, and in many diet-aid drugs.

Phenytoin

Brand Name: Dilantin®

Category Of Drug: Anticonvulsant

Intended Effects: To control epileptic seizures.

Side Effects: Slurred speech, confusion, dizziness, sleeplessness, mild nervousness, twitchings, headache, nausea, vomiting, constipation, measles-like rash, lupus, anemia, gum problems, excess facial hair, low blood sugar, liver problems.

Warnings: Discontinuation of this drug, even if replaced by another drug, should be done gradually, not suddenly. Is not recommended for seizures caused by blood sugar problems. Causes birth defects in animals — avoid during pregnancy. Known to be present in mothers' milk — avoid drug or avoid nursing. Is not adequate to control petit mal seizures.

Possible Interactions: Barbiturates may increase this drug's action. Blood thinners, antidepressants or alcohol may cause reduced effectiveness. People who are sensitive to hydantoin products should not take Dilantin®.

---

pHisoHex® (*Winthrop*)
See: Hexachlorophene

Phospholine Iodide® (*Ayerst*)
  See: Echothiophate

Pilocar® (*CooperVision*)
  See: Pilocarpine

Pilocarpine

Brand Names: Isopto Carpine®, Pilocar®

Category Of Drug: Antiglaucoma

Intended Effects: To control pressure within the eyeball-lin treating glaucoma.

Side Effects: Inflammation of the eyelids, headache, nearsightedness, reduced vision in poor light. Rare: retinal detachment. With long use: clouding of the lens.

Warnings: For use in the eye only. Should not be taken in cases of inflammation of the iris. Use caution when driving at night or doing other activities in poor light — vision may be reduced.

Pindolol
  See: Beta-Adrenergic Blocking Agent Class

Piroxicam

Brand Name: Feldene®

Category Of Drug: Anti-inflammatory, Fever Reducer, Pain Reliever, Anti-arthritis.

Intended Effects: To relieve the signs and symptoms of osteoarthritis and rheumatoid arthritis.

Side Effects: Most frequent (20%): Stomach or intestinal discomfort. Frequent (3-6%): upper abdominal distress or nausea. Less frequent (1-3%): loss of appetite, constipation, abdominal pain, diarrhea, indigestion, dizziness, vertigo, ringing in the ears, headache, "unwell" feeling, rash, fluid retention, vomiting, stomach or intestinal bleeding, ulcers, dry mouth, sweating, bruising, swollen eyes, blurred vision, eye irritation, general body pain, high blood pressure, low blood sugar, weight increase or decrease, depression, insomnia, nervousness. Rare (reported but unconfirmed): awareness of heartbeat, difficult breathing, uncontrolled muscles, difficult or painful urination.

Warnings: Do not use if aspirin or other anti-inflammatory drugs have caused bronchospasms, nasal growths or fluid retention around the heart. Use with caution in people with history of stomach or small intestine disease, impaired kidney or liver function, heart irregularities, high blood pressure or fluid retention.

Possible Interactions: May interact with some anticlotting drugs. Aspirin causes reduced effectiveness.

Polaramine® (*Schering*)
  See: Antihistamine Class

Polymox® (*Bristol*)
  See: Penicillin Class

Poly-Vi-Flor® (*Mead Johnson*)

Category Of Drug: Vitamins + Fluoride

Ingredients: Vitamins A + D + E + C + Thiamine + Ribo-flavin + Niacin + Pyridoxine + Cyanocobalamin + Fluoride

Intended Effects: To supplement the diet with essential vitamins, and to supplement the diet with fluoride to aid in the prevention of tooth decay in young children.

Side Effects: Rare: allergic rash.

Warnings: Tablets not for infants or children from birth to 2 years of age. Only for children ages 2-3 in areas where thedrinking water contains less than .3ppm of fluoride, or children over 3 where the drinking water contains .3-.7ppm of fluoride. Do not exceed recommended dosage.

Ponstel® (*Parke-Davis*)
  See: Mefenamic

Potassium Bicarbonate
  See: Potassium Supplement Class

Potassium Chloride

See: Potassium Supplement Class

Potassium Gluconate
See: Potassium Supplement Class

Potassium Supplement Class

Generic / Brand Names:
  Potassium Bicarbonate/K-Lyte®
  PotassiumChloride/Kay-ciel®,K-Lor®,Klotrix®,
  K- Tab®, Micro-K®,Slow-K®
  Potassium Gluconate/Kaon®

Category Of Drug: Mineral Supplement

Intended Effects: To supplement the body's supply of potassium, an essential electrolyte necessary for the contraction of the heart and the transmission of nerve impulses. (Depletion of potassium usually develops slowly as a consequence of taking diuretics, but supplementation may be required at other times as well.)

Side Effects: Nausea, abdominal discomfort, vomiting, diarrhea, mental confusion, tingling in the limbs, unusual tiredness or weakness, weakness of the legs, shortness of breath, difficult breathing. Rare: skin rash.

Warnings: Should be used with caution by people with kidney disease or impaired kidney function, people taking salt substitutes (which may already contain large amounts of potassium), people with heart disease or kidney obstruction. Diabetics and people with severe burns should use this drug with caution.

Possible Interactions: Sudden withdrawal from a potassium supplement can cause poisonous effects in people who have been taking digitalis. Salt substitutes such as "lite-salt" may contain large amounts of potassium, so dosage of potassium supplements should be adjusted. Spironolactone or triamterene, when taken with potassium supplements may cause an excessive rise in blood potassium levels which can be fatal.

Prazepam
  See: Benzodiazepine Class

Prazosin

Brand Name: Minipress®

Category Of Drug: Blood-Pressure Reducer

Intended Effects: To lower high blood pressure.

Side Effects: Frequent (5-10%): headache, drowsiness, lack of energy, weakness, pounding of the heart, nausea. Less frequent: vomiting, diarrhea, constipation, abdominal discomfort or pain, hives, shortness of breath, blackout, rapid heartbeat, nervousness, incoordinated movements, depression, tingling sensations, rash, itching, loss of hair, frequent urination, loss of bladder control, change in sex desire, blurred vision, red eyes, ringing in the ears, dry mouth, nasal congestion.

Warnings: Blood pressure may drop suddenly causing loss of consciousness.

Possible Interactions: This drug may increase the effects of other blood-pressure reducers.

Pred-Forte® Topical (*Allergan*)

Category Of Drug: Anti-inflammatory

Ingredients: Prednisolone + Polysorbate 80 + EDTA + Hydroxypropyl Methylcellulose + Benzalkonium Chloride

Intended Effects: To treat certain allergic and inflammatory conditions of the eye, to treat corneal injury caused by radiation, penetration of foreign bodies, chemical or heat burns, or certain non-pus-forming conjunctivitis. To treat herpes zoster (shingles) eye infections.

Side Effects: Blurred vision, drooping eyelids, seeing halos around lights, headache, eye pain, occasional stinging or burning. Viral and fungal infections of the cornea may become more severe. With long use: glaucoma, damage to optic nerves, other eye irregularities. Fungus infection may occur after use.

Warnings: Not for people with degenerative eye diseases, those with acute herpes simplex eye infections, tuberculosis of the eye, chicken pox, cow pox, or most other virus infections of the eye.

Prednisone
See: Adrenocorticoid Class - Systemic

Preludin® (*Boehringer*)

See: Appetite Suppressant Class

Premarin® (*Ayerst*)
  See: Estrogen Class - Systemic
  See: Estrogen Class-Vaginal

Primidone

Brand Name: Mysoline®

Category Of Drug: Anticonvulsant

Intended Effects: To treat certain epileptic seizures.

Side Effects: Incoordination, vertigo, nausea, loss of appetite, vomiting, fatigue, irritability, emotional disturbances, sexual impotency, drowsiness. Rare: megaloblastic anemia.

Warnings: Not for people with porphyria or people who are sensitive to phenobarbital. Do not discontinue this medication abruptly. Causes birth defects in animals — avoid during first three months of pregnancy. Known to be present in mothers' milk — avoid drug or avoid nursing. Drive and operate machinery with caution.

Possible Interactions: This drug taken with other anticonvulsants may alter seizure pattern — dosage adjustment may be necessary. Sedation may increase when taken with: tranquilizers, antihistamines, antidepressants, sedatives, sleep inducers, alcohol and narcotics.

Principen® (*Squibb*)

See: Penicillin Class

Pro-Banthine® (*Searle*)
See: Propantheline Bromide

Probenecid

Brand Name: Benemid®

Category Of Drug: Uric Acid Reducer, Anti-gout

Intended Effects: To treat gout and gouty arthritis. To increase the effect and duration of penicillin.

Side Effects: Headache, nausea, vomiting, frequent urination, sore gums, flushing, dizziness, anemia, hypersensitivity reactions. Development of kidney stones.

Warnings: Use with caution in patients with peptic ulcer. Not recommended to be used with penicillin or in patients with known kidney impairment. Treatment with Benemid® should not be started until an acute gouty attack has passed. Not for children under age two. Consult physician if acute gout attack occurs after therapy with this drug is started. Consult physician before discontinuing this drug.

Possible Interactions: Aspirin and aspirin-like drugs reduce the effectiveness of this drug. Interacts with sulfa drugs, indomethacin and thiazide diuretics.

Procainamide

Brand Names: Procan®-SR, Pronestryl®

Category Of Drug: Heart-Rhythm Regulator

Intended Effects: To regulate heart rhythm.

Side Effects: Lowered blood pressure. With large doses: reduced appetite, nausea, itching, bitter taste, weakness, diarrhea, mental depression, giddiness, hallucinations, psychosis, development of arthritis symptoms and facial rashes.

Warnings: Report to physician any soreness of mouth, gums or throat, unexplained fever or symptoms of upper respiratory tract infection. Not for people with myasthenia gravis. Should be used with caution by people with kidney or liver impairment or disease, those with lupus erythematosus, people taking any form of digitalis. People allergic to aspirin may also be allergic to this drug.

Possible Interactions: May increase the effects of blood-pressure reducers. May reduce the effects of certain drugs used to treat myasthenia gravis.

Procan® SR (*Parke-Davis*)
See: Procainamide

Procardia® (*Pfizer*)
See: Calcium Channel Inhibitors

Prochlorperazine
See: Phenothiazine Class

Progestin Class

Generic / Brand Names:
Medroxyprogesterone/Provera®
Norethindrone/Micronor®, Norlutate®
Norgestrel/Ovrette®

Category Of Drug: Female hormones

Intended Effects: To correct menstrual disorders caused by hormone imbalance, to prevent pregnancy, to test if the body is producing certain hormones, to treat certain forms of cancer in women.

Side Effects: Breast tenderness or flow from the nipples, rashes, itching, fluid retention, acne, loss of pigmentation, increased facial hair, increased clotting of the blood leading to the blockage of blood vessels, break-through bleeding, spotting, changes in menstrual flow, lack of menstruation, jaundice, mental depression, pre-cancerous changes in the cervix, high blood pressure, premenstrual tension, change in sexual desire, change in appetite, cystitis, headache, nervousness, dizziness, fatigue, backache, loss of scalp hair, weight change. Serious: thrombophlebitis (inflammation of a vein, usually in the legs, with the formation of a blood clot), stroke (blood clot and bleeding in the brain), pulmonary embolism (movement of blood clot to the lung), or retinal thrombosis (blood clot in blood vessels of the eye).

Warnings: Not for people with poor liver function, history of cancer of the genital organs or breast, abnormal and unexplained vaginal bleeding, or those with history of stroke, embolism, or thrombophlebitis. Causes birth defects — avoid during known or possible pregnancy. Known to be present in mothers' milk — avoid drug or avoid nursing. Should be used with caution by people with diabetes (because of decrease in glucose tolerance), by those with epilepsy, asthma, migraine headaches, history of mental depression, poor heart or kidney function. Sudden partial or complete loss of vision should be promptly reported to physician.

Possible Interactions: These drugs may increase the effects of phenothiazines. Antihistamines, phenylbutazone and phenobarbital may decrease the effects of these drugs.

Prolixin® (*Squibb*)
  See: Phenothiazine Class

Proloid® (*Parke-Davis*)
  See: Thyroid Hormone Class

Promethazine

Brand Name: Phenergan®

Category Of Drug: Antihistamine, Antivomiting, Sedative

Intended Effects: To relieve congestion during hay fever, allergies or colds; to control rashes, to reduce inflammation of the eyelids, to relieve allergic reactions to blood or plasma, to treat shock, to control nausea and vomiting associated with anesthesia in surgery, to help control pain, to treat and prevent motion sickness.

Side Effects: Infrequent: dryness of the mouth, blurred vision, drowsiness, dizziness. Rare: low white blood count and other blood disorders, increases and decreases in blood pressure, light sensitivity.

Warnings: May mask symptoms and diagnosis of other disease. Use alcohol with extreme caution. Because of possible drowsiness, drive and operate machinery with caution.

Possible Interactions: Sedation may increase when taken with: tranquilizers, antihistamines, antidepressants, sedatives, sleep inducers, alcohol and narcotics.

Pronestyl® (*Squibb*)
  See: Procainamide

Propantheline Bromide

Brand Name: Pro-Banthine®

Category Of Drug: Antispasm

Intended Effects: To treat peptic ulcer, to relieve discomfort from excessive activity and spasm of digestive tract.

Side Effects: Blurred vision, dryness of mouth or throat, constipation, urinary hesitancy, rapid or pounding heartbeat, loss of sense of taste, nervousness, headache, drowsiness, mental confusion, dizziness, insomnia, nausea, vomiting, bloated feeling, skin rash, hives, decreased sweating. In the eyes: dilation of pupils which can lead to light sensitivity, increased pressure in the eyeball.

Warnings: Should be used with caution in the elderly, and by people with myasthenia gravis, high blood pressure, coronary heart disease, congestive heart failure, kidney or liver disease, open-angle glaucoma, enlarged prostate gland, history of peptic ulcer disease, overactive thyroid. Not for patients who cannot empty the bladder completely, those with severe ulcerative colitis, narrow-angle glaucoma, those whose stomachs do not empty completely into the intestine, or those with blurred vision. May cause drowsiness — drive and operate machinery with caution. Use caution in hot weather because of the possibility of heat stroke from decreased sweating.

Possible Interactions: If this drug is taken with slow-dissolving tablets of digoxin, increased serum digoxin levels may result. May delay the absorption of other medication taken with it at the same time. Tricyclic antidepressants, phenothiazines, quinidine or procainamide, MAO inhibitors, haloperidol, and antihistamines may intensify certain side effects if used with this drug. Sedation may increase when taken with: tranquilizers, antihistamines, antidepressants, sedatives, sleep inducers, alcohol and narcotics.

Propine® (*Allergan*)
See: Dipivefrin

Propoxyphene

Brand Name: Darvon®

Category Of Drug: Narcotic, Pain Reliever

Intended Effects: To relieve mild to moderate pain.

Side Effects: Dizziness, nausea and vomiting (which may be reduced by lying down). Drowsiness, constipation, abdominal pain, skin rash, lightheadedness, headache, weakness, minor visual disturbances, feelings of elation or discomfort, liver problems.

Warnings: Not for suicidal or addiction-prone people. Known to be present in mothers' milk — avoid drug or avoid nursing. Do not exceed recommended dosage — psychological and physical dependence may occur. Drive and operate machinery with caution. Not for children under 12.

Possible Interactions: Sedation may increase when taken with tranquilizers, sleep inducers, antihistamines, antidepressants, sedatives, alcohol and narcotics.

Propranolol
See: Beta-Adrenergic Blocking Agent Class

Proventil® (*Schering*)
See: Albuterol

Provera® (*Upjohn*)
See: Progestin Class

Pseudoephedrine

Brand Names: Novafed®, Sudafed®

Category Of Drug: Decongestant

Intended Effects: To relieve nasal congestion caused by the common cold, hay fever, sinus inflammation and allergies.

Side Effects: Nervousness, insomnia, headache, dizziness, skin rash.

Warnings: Reduce dosage if nervousness, nausea, headache, sleeplessness or dizziness occur. People with high blood pressure, heart disease, diabetes, glaucoma, thyroid disease or urinary retention should use this drug only under advice of physician. Known to be present in mothers' milk — avoid drug or avoid nursing.

Possible Interactions: Many over-the-counter drugs for colds, allergies and coughs react unfavorably with this drug. MAO inhibitors, tricyclic antidepressants, and ergot-related preparations may cause a dangerous increase in blood pressure. Phenytoin may cause serious problems with heart rhythm.

Psyllium
  See: Laxatives-Bulk Class

Pyridium® (*Parke-Davis*)
See: Phenazopyridine

Quibron® (*Mead Johnson*)
  See: Guaifenesin
  See: Theophylline

Quinaglute® (*Berlex*)
See: Quinidine

Quinamm™ (*Merrell Dow*)

Category Of Drug: Muscle Relaxant

Ingredients: Quinine

Intended Effects: To prevent or treat night time leg muscle cramps associated with arthritis, varicose veins, diabetes, thrombophlebitis, hardening of the arteries, and certain foot deformities.

Side Effects: Ringing in the ears, severe headaches, dizziness, stomach distress, fever, deafness, visual disturbances, skin rash, blood platelet deficiency, confusion, restlessness, apprehension, sweating or flushing of the face.

Warnings: Not for patients with ringing in the ears, inflammation of optic nerve, history of blackwater fever, or G-6-PD enzyme deficiency. Take this drug with or after meals to minimize possible stomach upset. Causes birth defects in animals — avoid during pregnancy. Known to be present in mothers' milk — avoid drug or avoid nursing.

Possible Interactions: May increase the action of warfarin and other oral anticlotting drugs. Antacids containing aluminum may cause delayed or decreased absorption.

Quinidex Extentabs® (*Robins*)
See: Quinidine

Quinidine

Brand Name: Quinaglute®, Quinidex Extentabs®

Category Of Drug: Heart-Rhythm Regulator

Intended Effects: To correct certain heart rhythm disorders by slowing and regulating the heartbeat.

Side Effects: Ringing in the ears, headache, nausea, disturbed vision, disruption of heart rhythm, ballooning of arteries, vomiting, stomach pain, diarrhea, anemia and other blood disorders, bleeding under the skin, fever, loss of balance, apprehension, excitement, confusion, light sensitivity, night blindness, pain in the eyes, reddening and itching of the skin, hive-like rash within the throat, shock, difficult breathing, cessation of breathing.

Warnings: Known to be present in mothers' milk — avoid drug or avoid nursing.

Possible Interactions: Effects are increased by potassium. May interact with digitalis medicines to cause very slow heart beat. Use nicotine with caution as it may alter the heart's pattern and mask quinidine's effects.

Ranitidine

Brand Name: Zantac®

Category Of Drug: Stomach Acid Secretion Inhibitor

Intended Effects: To treat active duodenal ulcers by

reducing the flow of stomach acid and allowing ulcers to heal.

Side Effects: Most frequent (3%): headache. Rare (less than 1%): "unwell" feelings, dizziness, constipation, nausea, abdominal pain, rash. Very rare: decrease in white blood cell and platelet count, hepatitis.

Warnings: Dose should be adjusted in people with impaired kidney function. Caution should be used in people with liver diseases. Known to be present in mothers' milk — avoid drug or avoid nursing.

Note: This drug is claimed to have fewer side effects and interactions than cimetidine, a drug with similar action.

Rauwolfia Alkaloid Class

Generic/Brand Names:
Deserpidine/Enduronyl®
Rauwolfia Serpentina/ Rauzide®
Reserpine/Demi-Regroton®, Diupres®, Hydropres®,
  Regroton®,Regroton®, salutensin®, Ser-Ap-Es®,

Category Of Drug: Tranquilizer, Blood-Pressure Reducer

Intended Effects: To reduce high blood pressure, to relieve symptoms of agitated psychotic states (schizophrenia).

Side Effects: Drowsiness, tiredness, nasal stuffiness, dry mouth, acid indigestion, diarrhea, nausea, intestinal cramps, depression, changes in menstrual schedule, water retention, reddening of the eyes, glaucoma, skin rash, headache, dizziness, breast enlargement, nightmares, deafness, weight gain, loss of appetite, insomnia, loss of sex drive.

Warnings: Extreme caution should be used in treating patients with mental depression with this drug. Should be used cautiously by people with peptic ulcer, gallstones, ulcerative colitis, or impaired kidney function. Dosage may need to be adjusted in hot weather because of altered blood pressure. Use machinery and drive with caution. Causes birth defects in animals — avoid during pregnancy. Known to be present in mothers' milk — avoid drug or avoid nursing.

Possible Interactions: If taken with digitalis, this drug may cause heart rhythm disturbances. MAO inhibitors should be avoided or used with extreme caution, to avoid severe depression. Sedation may increase when taken with: tranquilizers, antihistamines, antidepressants, sedatives, sleep inducers, alcohol and narcotics.

Rauzide® (*Squibb*)
  See: Rauwolfia Alkaloid Class
  See: Thiazide Diuretic Class

Reglan® (*Robins*)
  See: Metoclopramide

Regroton® (*USV*)
  See: Rauwolfia Alkaloid Class

Reserpine
 See: Rauwolfia Alkaloid Class

Restoril® (*Sandoz*)
 See: Temazepam

Retin-A® (*Ortho*)
 See: Tretinoin

Ridaura® (*Smith Kline & French*)
 See: Auranofin

Ritalin® (*CIBA*)
 See: Methylphenidate

Robaxin® (*Robins*)
 See: Methocarbamol

Robaxisal® (*Robins*)
 See: Methocarbamol
 See: Salicylates

Robicillin VK (*Robins*)
 See: Penicillin Class

Robitet® (*Robins*)
  See: Tetracycline Class

Robitussin® (*Robins*)
  See: Guaifenesin

Note: No Rx prescription required

Robitussin A-C® (*Robins*)
  See: Guaifenesin
  See: Codeine

Robitussin-DM® (*Robins*)
  See: Guaifenesin
  See: Dextromethorphan

Note: No Rx prescription required

Rondec™ (*Ross*)
  See: Antihistamine Class
  See: Pseudoephedrine

Note: Rondec T™ = Tablet form
Rondec S™ = Syrup form
Rondec D™ = drops

Rondec-DM™ (*Ross*)

Category Of Drug: Antihistamine, Decongestant, Anti-cough

Ingredients: Carbinoxamine + Pseudoephedrine + Dextromethorphan

Intended Effects: To provide relief for symptoms of the common cold, stuffy or runny nose, coughing, bronchitis or chest congestion.

Side Effects: Sleepiness, dizziness, vomiting, nausea, dry mouth, headache, nervousness, loss of appetite, heartburn, weakness, stomach upset, depression, breathing difficulties, increased heart rate or blood pressure, tremors, lack of sleep. Rare: convulsions, excitability in children.

Warnings: Use with caution in elderly patients or those with high blood pressure, heart disease, asthma, over-active thyroid or diabetes. Drive or operate machinery with caution.

Possible Interactions: Avoid alcohol and central nervous system depressants. May increase the effects of tricyclic antidepressants and barbiturates. May reduce the effectiveness of reserpine, methyldopa, mecamylamine and narcotics. MAO inhibitors increase the drying effects of this drug.

Rufen® (*Boots*)
  See: Ibuprofen

Ru-Tuss® (*Boots*)

272

Category Of Drug: Antihistamine, Nasal Decongestant

Ingredients: Phenylephrine + Phenylpropanolamine + Chlorpheniramine + Hyoscyamine + Atropine + Scopolamine

Intended Effects: To relieve symptoms of sinus, nasal and upper respiratory tract irritation and congestion.

Side Effects: Rash, drowsiness, giddiness, tightness of the chest, dry mouth and throat, thickening of bronchial secretions, frequent urination, higher or lower blood pressure, fainting, dizziness, ringing in the ears, headache, incoordinated movements, visual disturbances, loss of appetite, nausea, vomiting, diarrhea, constipation, nervousness, inability to sleep, rapid or pounding heartbeat.

Warnings: May cause drowsiness — use extreme caution while driving or operating machinery. Should be used with caution by people with urinary bladder neck obstruction, high blood pressure, heart disease, glaucoma, or enlarged thyroid. Not for people with bronchial asthma or those who are allergic to antihistamines or bronchial tube relaxers. Not for children under the age of 12.

Possible Interactions: Do not take with MAO inhibitors. Sedation may increase when taken with: tranquilizers, antihistamines, antidepressants, sedatives, sleep inducers, alcohol and narcotics.

Ru-Vert 2® (*Reed-Rowell*)
See: Meclizine

Rynatan® *(Wallace)*

Category Of Drug: Antihistamine, Decongestant

Ingredients: Phenylephrine + Chlorpheniramine + Pyrilamine

Intended Effects: To relieve nasal congestion (stuffy nose) associated with sinus infection, the common cold, allergies and other upper respiratory tract conditions.

Side Effects: Excitation, drowsiness, sedation, dryness of nose and throat. In elderly patients: dizziness, sedation or low blood pressure.

Warnings: Use with caution in patients with high blood pressure, heart or blood vessel disease, overactive thyroid, narrow-angle glaucoma, diabetes or enlarged prostate. Drive and operate machinery with caution while taking this drug. May cause birth defects in animals — avoid during first three months of pregnancy or use with caution. May be present in mothers' milk — avoid drug or avoid nursing.

Possible Interactions: Sedation may increase when taken with: tranquilizers, antihistamines, antidepressants, sedatives, sleep inducers, alcohol and narcotics.

Salicylate Class

Generic/Brand Names:
Aspirin/Ecotrin®
Buffered Aspirin/Ascriptin®
Choline Salicylate + Magnesium Salicylate/Trilisate®

Salsalate/Disalcid®

Category Of Drug: Pain Reliever, Fever Reducer, Anti-inflammatory, Anticlotting.

Intended Effects: To reduce pain, fever, inflammation and blood clotting. To relieve symptoms of arthritis. Buffering (if present with aspirin) may reduce the chance of upset stomach.

Side Effects: Mild drowsiness, hives, upset stomach, runny nose, heartburn, vomiting, nausea, skin rash, activation of peptic ulcer, increased tendency to bleed. Reduced production of blood cells, kidney damage from long use or large doses.

Warnings: Avoid if sensitive to aspirin or acetaminophen. Avoid if bleeding problems exist. Nursing mothers and pregnant women, especially in the last trimester, should avoid aspirin. Should be discontinued at least one week before surgery.

Possible Interactions: May increase the effects of antidiabetic drugs and insulin, anticlotting drugs, adrenocorticoids, penicillins, methotrexate and phenytoin. May decrease the effects of allopurinol, certain gout medications, and spironolactone. Vitamin C in large doses taken as ascorbic acid may cause poisonous reaction. Antacids, phenobarbital, propranolol and reserpine may cause decreased effects. Adrenocorticoids, furosemide, phenylbutazone, indomethacin and para-aminosalicylic acid, if taken with salicylates, should be monitored by physician. Butazones, adrenocorticoids, or alcohol may increase the risk of stomach or intestinal ulcers.

Note: Many salicylates, such as aspirin, are

275

available without prescription.

Salsalate

Brand Name: Disalcid®

Category Of Drug: Anti-inflammatory, Pain Reliever, Fever-Reducer

Intended Effects: To relieve swelling, pain and fever of rheumatoid arthritis, osteoarthritis and other related rheumatic disorders.

Side Effects: Temporary hearing loss, nausea, heartburn, ringing in the ears, indigestion. Overdose: headache, drowsiness, vomiting or diarrhea, strong ringing in the ears.

Warnings: Not for people sensitive to salicylates. Should be used with caution by people with chronic kidney problems or peptic ulcers. Causes birth defects in animals — avoid during pregnancy.

Possible Interactions: Increases the effects of anticlotting agents.

Salutensin® *(Bristol)*
  See: Rauwolfia Alkaloid Class
  See: Thiazide Diuretic Class

Secobarbital
  See: Barbiturate Class

Seconal® *(Lilly)*
  See: Barbiturate Class

Sectral® *(Wyeth)*
  See: Beta-Adrenergic Blocking Agent Class

Seldane® *(Merrell Dow)*
  See: Terfenadine

Selsun® *(Abbott)*

Category Of Drug: Anti-dandruff

Ingredients: Selenium Sulfide

Intended Effects: To treat dandruff or excessive oiliness of the scalp.

Side Effects: Oiliness or dryness of hair and scalp, increased hair loss, discoloration of hair, (which may be minimized or avoided with thorough rinsing), skin irritation.

Warnings: Avoid contact with the eyes. Do not use if blistered, oozing or raw areas exist on the scalp. Do not use more frequently than needed to maintain control. May damage jewelry — remove jewelry before use.

Senna
  See: Laxative-Stimulant Class

Senokot® (*Purdue Frederick*)
  See: Laxative-Stimulant Class

Note: No Rx prescription required

Septra® (*Burroughs Wellcome*)
  See: Sulfonamide Class-Systemic

SER-AP-ES® (*CIBA*)
  See: Rauwolfia Alkaloid Class
  See: Hydralazine
  See: Thiazide Diuretic Class

Serax® (*Wyeth*)
  See: Benzodiazepine Class

Silvadene® (*Marion*)

Category Of Drug: Anti-infective

Ingredient: Silver Sulfadiazine

Intended Effects: To treat and prevent infection of second and third degree burns.

Side Effects: Since patients with severe burns are treated with several therapeutic agents at one time, it is difficult to determine which of the reported side effects occurred from this drug. Most frequent (2-5%): burning, rash or itching.

Frequent: increased sensitivity of the skin to sunlight, rash, or itching. Infrequent: pale skin, sore throat, unusual bleeding or bruising, difficulty in swallowing, unexplained fever, aching of muscles of joints, yellowing of skin or eyes.

Warnings: Should not be used on premature or newborn infants.

Possible Interactions: People allergic to other sulfonamides may also be allergic to this drug.

Sinemet® (*Merck Sharp & Dohme*)

Category Of Drug: Antitremor

Ingredients: Carbidopa + Levodopa

Intended Effects: To reduce the tremors, sluggish movements, walking disturbances and rigidity of Parkinson's disease.

Side Effects: Uncontrolled or unusual body movements of the tongue, face, hands, arms, head and upper body. Mental depression, mental or mood changes, nausea, dry mouth, dizziness, fainting, irregular heartbeats, vomiting, difficult urination. Rare: hemolytic anemia, high blood pressure, duodenal ulcer, phlebitis, loss of appetite, gastrointestinal bleeding.

Warnings: Causes birth defects in animals — avoid during first three months of pregnancy. May be present in mothers' milk — avoid drug or avoid nursing. May be taken with food to minimize stomach upset. Should be used with caution by people with severe heart, lung or blood vessel disease, bronchial asthma, kidney or liver disease, or people with history of peptic ulcer, melanoma, convulsive disorders, narrow-angle glaucoma, diabetes, psychotic states, or those with lingering heart irregularities after a heart attack.

Possible Interactions: Levodopa must be discontinued before this drug is started. If taken with blood-pressure reducers, excessive lowering of the blood pressure may result. Reserpine, phenytoin, papaverine, butyrophenones, benzodiazepines and phenothiazines may decrease the effects of this drug. Do not take within 14 days of MAO inhibitors. Avoid vitamins with B6 because they decrease its effectiveness.

Sinequan® (*Roerig*)
  See: Tricyclic Antidepressant Class

Singlet® (*Merrell Dow*)

Category Of Drug: Decongestant, Antihistamine, Pain Reliever

Ingredients: Phenylephrine + Chlorpheniramine + Acetaminophen

Intended Effects: To relieve congestion of nose, sinuses and throat due to colds, allergies or infections.

Side Effects: Dryness of throat and nose, drowsiness, restlessness, dizziness, loss of appetite, nausea, headache, weakness, blurred vision, nervousness, tremor, rapid or pounding heartbeat, fear, anxiety, insomnia, hallucinations or convulsions.

Warnings: Causes birth defects in animals — avoid during first three months of pregnancy. Not recommended for people with severe high blood pressure, severe coronary artery disease, people with peptic ulcer, glaucoma or high intra-eye pressure, urinary retention, impaired kidney or liver function, asthma attack. Not for children under 12. Should be used with extreme caution by people with diabetes, coronary heart disease, overactive thyroid, enlarged prostate. Drive and operate machinery with caution.

Possible Interactions: If taken with MAO inhibitors, excessive rise in blood pressure may result. Beta-blockers increase the effects of this drug. May reduce the blood pressure lowering effect of methyldopa, mecamylamine, reserpine and veratrum alkaloids. Sedation may increase when taken with: tranquilizers, antihistamines, antidepressants, sedatives, sleep inducers, alcohol and narcotics.

Slo-Phyllin® (*Rorer*)
  See: Xanthine Class

Slow-K® (*CIBA*)
  See: Potassium Supplement Class

Soma® (*Wallace*)
  See: Carisoprodol

Sorbitrate® (*Stuart*)
  See: Nitrate Class

Spectrobid® (*Roerig*)
See: Penicillin Class

Spironolactone

Brand Name: Aldactone®

Intended Effects: To relieve fluid retention, to lower blood pressure; often prescribed for patients with congestive heart failure, cirrhosis of the liver, certain kidney problems, high blood pressure, or deficient potassium levels in their blood; helps flush excess amounts of water and sodium (salt) from the system, while not reducing potassium levels.

Side Effects: May cause electrolyte imbalances, dry mouth and throat, lethargy, drowsiness, breast enlargement, mild acidosis, stomach distress, headache, confusion, menstrual irregularities, excess hair growth.

Warnings: Normally, potassium supplements should not be taken with this drug. Should not be used by patients having certain severe kidney problems or having high levels of potassium in their blood. Known to be present in mothers' milk — avoid drug or avoid nursing. Salt intake should be checked by a physician.

Possible Interactions: May increase the action of other blood-pressure reducers; large doses of aspirin may decrease this drug's effectiveness. Do not take with triamterene. This drug may decrease the effects of anticlotting drugs and digitalis.

Stelazine® (*Smith Kline & French*)
  See: Phenothiazine Class

Stilphostrol® (*Miles*)
  See: Estrogen Class-Systemic

Stuartnatal® 1+1 (*Stuart*)

Category Of Drug: Vitamin/Mineral Supplement

Ingredients: Vitamins A + C + D + E + Folic Acid + Thiamine + Riboflavin + Niacin + B6 + B12 + Calcium + Iodine + Iron + Magnesium

Intended Effects: To supplement the mothers' vitamin intake during pregnancy and breast-feeding.

Side Effects: Yellow dye #5, which is present in this preparation, may cause allergic reactions, including bronchial asthma, in certain people, especially those sensitive to aspirin. This dye provokes an allergic reaction in only a small percentage of the population.

Warnings: Taking vitamins including folic acid may mask the symptoms of pernicious anemia.

Sucralfate

Brand Name: Carafate®

Category Of Drug: Anti-ulcer

Intended Effects: To treat duodenal ulcers. (short-term treatment only).

Side Effects: Constipation, diarrhea, nausea, gastric discomfort, indigestion, dry mouth, rash, itching, back pain, dizziness, sleepiness, loss of balance.

Warnings: Should only be used for short-term (up to 8 weeks) treatment of duodenal ulcers. Should be taken on an empty stomach; one hour before meals or two hours after meals. Should be taken for the complete length of time prescribed.

Possible Interactions: Antacids may be used but not within one-hour of taking sucralfate. May reduce the effects of tetracycline, phenytoin, digoxin, or cimetidine if taken within two hours of sucralfate. May reduce or alter the effects of any other drug. Other drugs should be prescribed with care.

Sudafed® (*Burroughs Wellcome*)
  See: Pseudoephedrine

Note: No Rx prescription required

Sulamyd® (*Schering*)
  See: Sulfonamide Class-Topical

Sulfacetamide
  See: Sulfonamide Class-Topical

Sulfa Drugs

See: Sulfonamide Class-Systemic
See: Sulfonamide Class-Topical

Sulfamethoxazole

See: Sulfonamide Class-Systemic

Sulfamethoxazole + Trimethoprim

See: Sulfonamide Class-Systemic
See: Sulfonamide Class-Topical

Sulfinpyrazone

Brand Name: Anturane®

Category Of Drug: Uric Acid Reducer, Anti-gout

Intended Effects: To reduce the frequency and severity of gout attacks. Not intended for treatment of acute gout attacks. To reduce the severity of recurring heart attacks, to regulate the uric acid content of the urine. To reduce the tendency to form blood clots.

Side Effects: Development of kidney stones, nausea, abdominal pain, vomiting, skin rashes, fatigue, fever, sore throat, unusual bleeding, bruising, stomach or intestinal bleeding.

Warnings: Should be taken with food or drink to reduce stomach irritation. During early stages of treatment, this drug may cause acute attacks from kidney stones or gout.

Avoid aspirin and other salicylate products since these may cause unusual bleeding. Consult physician before discontinuing. Peptic ulcer, colitis, or duodenal ulcer patients should be closely monitored by physician, since unusual bleeding is possible. Periodic blood counts and kidney function studies are recommended.

Possible Interactions: May increase the effects of anticlotting drugs, aspirin, sulfa drugs, penicillin, insulin and certain antidiabetic drugs. May decrease the effects of oral contraceptives. Aspirin may decrease its effects. Probenecid may increase its effectiveness in treatment of chronic gout.

Sulfisoxazole

See: Sulfonamide Class-Systemic
See: Sulfonamide Class-Topical

Sulfonamide Class-Systemic

Generic/Brand Names:
Sulfamethoxazole/Gantanol®
Sulfamethoxazole.Trimethoprim/Bactrim®,
    Bactrim®DS, Septra®, Septra®DS
Sulfisoxazole/Gantrisin®

Category Of Drug: Anti-infective

Intended Effects: To help the body combat infections.

Side Effects: Blood disorders, including anemia and bleeding under the skin. Skin rashes, destruction of the skin, serum sickness, itching, shock, fluid retention around the eye, light sensitivity, inflammation of the joints and heart, nausea, stomach pain, hepatitis, diarrhea, inflammation of the pancreas, headache, pains in the limbs, depression, convulsions, heart disorders, hallucinations, ringing in the ears, loss of balance, insomnia, apathy, fatigue, muscle weakness, nervousness, fever, chills, inflammation of arteries, swelling of the thyroid gland, loss of body fluids and low blood sugar levels.

Warnings: Causes birth defects in animals — avoid during first three months of pregnancy. Known to be present in mothers' milk — avoid drug or avoid nursing. Take with caution in people with poor kidney or liver function. Insure large intake of water to produce adequate volume of dilute urine. Some sulfonamides may cause sensitivity to sun. After treatment with sulfonamides vitamin C supplement may be needed. Watch for sore throat, paleness or jaundice (yellow skin) which may indicate serious blood disorders.

Possible Interactions: May decrease effects of penicillin. Aspirin may increase effects of sulfonamides. Methenamine when taken with sulfonamides may cause dangerous crystallization and loss of kidney function. When taken with MAO inhibitors, serious anemia may result. Bleeding may result when taken with anticlotting drugs. There is a potential for hypoglycemia (low blood sugar) when taken with antidiabetics.

Sulfonamide Class-Topical

Brand Names: AVC® Vaginal Cream, Gantrisin® — Ophthalmic, Sulamyd® Ophthalmic, Sultrin® Vaginal Cream.

Category Of Drug: Anti-infective

Intended Effects: To help combat infections in the eye or vagina.

Side Effects: Itching, redness, rash, swelling, or burning.

Warnings: Use cautiously by those who are sensitive to other sulfonamides, sulfones, diuretics, sulfonylureas, carbonic anhydrase inhibitors or furosemide. Vaginally: use of tampons not recommended, continue full course of treatment, even if menstruating. Administer medication properly, especially during pregnancy. May stain clothing. In cases of vaginal infections, sexual partner may need treatment — use of condom advised.

Possible Interactions: May interact with eye medicines containing silver.

Sulindac

Brand Name: Clinoril®

Category Of Drug: Anti-inflammatory, Anti-arthritic

Intended Effects: To relieve immediate or long-term symptoms of osteoarthritis, rheumatoid arthritis, gouty arthritis, bursitis.

Side Effects: Stomach ache, nausea, vomiting, constipation, diarrhea, rash, dizziness, headache, nervousness, ringing in the ears, liver or pancreas problems.

Warnings: People with ulcer problems should be carefully watched by physician. May cause abnormal liver function tests. Should be used cautiously by patients with serious heart, blood pressure, or fluid retention problems. Not for people who are sensitive to this product or those for whom aspirin or other non-adrenocorticoid anti-inflammatory drugs may cause asthma attacks. Do not discontinue this drug suddenly.

Possible Interactions: May increase the effects of some anticlotting drugs, sulfonamides, or medicine for diabetes. Alcohol may increase the risk of stomach bleeding. Aspirin and phenobarbital may decrease its effectiveness.

Sultrin® (*Ortho*)
  See: Sulfonamide Class-Topical

Sumycin® (*Squibb*)
  See: Tetracycline Class

Suprofen

Brand Name: Suprol®

Category Of Drug: Anti-inflammatory, Pain Reliever, Fever Reducer

Intended Effects: To relieve mild to moderate pain; to relieve menstrual cramps.

Side Effects: Most frequent (1-15%): nausea, indigestion, loose stools, diarrhea, upset stomach, abdominal pain, constipation, vomiting, flatulence, stomach bleeding, inflammation of the lining of the stomach, headache, dizziness, sleepiness, mood changes, sleep disturbances, tingling sensations, body pains, weakness, loss of strength, water retention, congestion, high blood pressure, awareness of heartbeat, skin irritation, itching, skin rash, urinary frequency, difficult urination, pus in the urine, muscle cramps, bursitis, changes in vision, ringing in the ears, pink eye. Less frequent (less than 1%): allergic reactions, reduction of blood hemoglobin, difficult breathing, peptic ulcers, inflammation of the stomach and the intestine, nosebleed, appetite changes, inflammation of the kidney. Rare (reported but unconfirmed): jaundice, increased heart rate, lime green urine, reduction in the number of platelets in the blood.

Warnings: Should be used with great caution by people with gastrointestinal bleeding, peptic ulcers, poor kidney function, low blood hemoglobin, fluid retention, high blood pressure, history of heart failure or liver problems, in people with stomach or kidney disease, by the elderly, and people taking diuretics. Should not be given to people in whom aspirin or other non-steroidal anti-inflammatory drugs cause bronchospasm, hives, nettles's rash, inflammation of the mucous membranes of the nose, or other sensitivity reactions. Should be taken with antacids, food or drink to reduce stomach irritation. Bleeding time may be prolonged when taking this medicine. May cause birth defects — avoid during last three months of pregnancy. Known to be present in mothers' milk — avoid drug or avoid nursing. People on anticlotting or antidiabetic drugs should be closely monitored.

Possible Interactions: May react with anticlotting or antidiabetic drugs. May increase the bleeding time when taken with anticlotting drugs.

Suprol® (*McNeil Pharmaceuticals*)
  See: Suprofen

Surfak® (*Hoechst-Roussel*)
  See: Laxative-Emollient Class

Note: No Rx prescription required

Symmetrel® (*Du Pont*)
  See: Amantadine

Synalar® (*Syntex*)
  See: Adrenocorticoid Class-Topical

Synalgos®-DC (*Wyeth*)

Category Of Drug: Pain Reliever, Sedative

Ingredients: Dihydrocodeine + Promethazine + Aspirin + Caffeine

Intended Effects: To relieve moderate to moderately severe pain while providing sedation.

Side Effects: Lightheadedness, dizziness, drowsiness, sedation, nausea, vomiting, constipation, itching. Rare: low blood pressure.

Warnings: Use with extreme caution by people with

peptic ulcer or poor blood clotting. Tolerance dependence, or addition may develop after repeated use. People who have had a sensitivity reaction to phenothiazines should not take this drug. Drive and operate machinery with caution. Should be used with caution by people with heart, blood vessel or liver disease, the elderly, those with underactive thyroid, Addison's disease, enlarged prostate and difficulties in urination.

Possible Interactions: May cause bleeding when taken with anticlotting drugs. Sedation may increase when taken with: tranquilizers, antihistamines, antidepressants, sedatives, sleep inducers, alcohol and narcotics.

Synthroid® (*Flint*)
See: Thyroid Hormone Class

Tagamet® (*Smith Kline & French*)
See: Cimetidine

Talwin® (*Winthrop*)
See: Pentazocine

Talwin® Compound (*Winthrop*)
See: Pentazocine
See: Salicylate Class

Tavist® (*Dorsey*)
See: Antihistamine Class

Tedral® (*Parke-Davis*)

Category Of Drug: Bronchial-Tube Relaxer

Ingredients: Theophylline + Ephedrine + Phenobarbital

Intended Effects: To treat asthma.

Side Effects: Drowsiness, mild stomach distress, pounding heartbeat, insomnia, tremors, difficulty in urination, and central nervous system stimulation.

Warnings: Drowsiness may occur — drive and operate machinery with caution. Not for people with porphyria. May be habit-forming. Use with caution in people with heart disease, severe high blood pressure, enlarged prostate, overactive thyroid, or glaucoma. This drug is more effective if taken on an empty stomach — however, if stomach upset occurs, the drug may be taken with or after meals. Use with caution in children under the age of 2. Avoid alcohol.

Possible Interactions: Sedation may increase when taken with: tranquilizers, antihistamines, antidepressants, sedatives, sleep inducers, alcohol and narcotics.

Tegopen® (*Bristol*)
See: Penicillin Class

Tegretol® (*Geigy*)
See: Carbamazepine

Teldrin® (*Smith Kline & French*)
  See: Antihistamine Class

Note: No Rx prescription required

Temaril® (*Smith Kline & French*)
  See: Trimeprazine

Temazepam

Brand Name: Restoril®

Category Of Drug: Sleeping Aid

Intended Effects: To relieve insomnia or difficulty in sleeping.

Side Effects: Most common (17%): drowsiness. Frequent (2-7%): dizziness, lethargy, confusion, euphoria, relaxed feeling. Less frequent (1-2%): weakness, loss of appetite, diarrhea. Rare (less than 1%): tremor, lack of concentration, awareness of heartbeat, loss of balance, hallucinations, excitement, stimulation, and excessive activity.

Warnings: Causes birth defects in animals — avoid during pregnancy. Should be used with caution in the elderly, in those with impaired kidney or liver function, narrow-angle glaucoma, history of drug dependence or abuse, or people with severe chronic obstructive heart disease. Drive or operate machinery with caution if drowsiness or dizziness occurs. Should be used with extreme caution by severely depressed people. High doses taken over a long period of time may produce psychological or physical dependence. Discontinue gradually after prolonged therapy to avoid withdrawal symptoms. Not for use by children.

Possible Interactions: Sedation may increase when taken with: tranquilizers, antihistamines, antidepressants, sedatives, sleep inducers, alcohol and narcotics.

Tenormin® (*Stuart*)
  See: Beta-Adrenergic Blocking Agent Class

Tenuate® (*Merrell Dow*)
  See: Appetite Suppressant Class

Terbutaline

Brand Name: Brethine®

Category Of Drug: Bronchial-Tube Relaxer

Intended Effects: To relieve breathing difficulties caused by bronchial asthma or emphysema.

Side Effects: Nervousness, tremors, headache, increased heart rate, pounding heartbeat, drowsiness, nausea, vomiting, sweating, muscle cramps. (Many of these side effects should diminish as use of drug continues.)

Warnings: Should not be used by people known to be sensitive to sympathomimetic amines. Should be used with caution by pregnant or nursing women, or patients with diabetes, high blood pressure, heart disease, over-active thyroid or problems with seizures. Should not be used in children under 12. Do not use if allergic to other bronchial-tube relaxers.

Possible Interactions: Avoid taking with epinephrine or MAO inhibitors. Propranolol may decrease the effectiveness of this drug.

Terfenadine

Brand Name: Seldane®

Category Of Drug: Antihistamine

Intended Effects: To relieve symptoms of allergies, including sneezing, runny nose, itching and watery eyes.

Side Effects: Headache, drowsiness, fatigue, dry mouth, sore throat, nausea, stuffy nose, cough, dizziness, vomiting, upset stomach, itching, dry nose, nervousness, dry throat, increased appetite, weakness. Infrequent: hair loss, allergic attack, fluid retention around the heart, difficult breathing, depression, milk secreted from nipples, insomnia, menstrual disorders, muscle pain, nightmares, awareness of heartbeat, tingling sensations, sweating, increased heart rate, tremors, frequent urination, visual disturbances.

Warnings: Should be stored in a tightly closed container in a cool, dry place away from heat or direct sunlight. Because of terfenadine's drying effects, it should be used with caution in people with diseases in the lower respiratory system.

Possible Interactions: None known.

Terpin Hydrate + Codeine

Category Of Drug: Anticough, Phlegm Loosener

Intended Effects: To suppress coughing.

Side Effects: Nausea, stomach pain, vomiting, drowsiness.

See: Codeine

Tetracycline Class

Generic / Brand Names:
Doxycycline/Vibramycin®, Vibratabs®
Minocycline/Minocin®
Tetracycline/Achromycin®,Panmycin®,Robitet®,
    Sumycin®

Category Of Drug: Antibiotic

Intended Effects: To combat infections.

Side Effects: Loss of appetite, nausea, vomiting, diarrhea, difficulty in swallowing, colon inflammation, fungus infections, especially in the region of the anus and genitals, rashes (including light-sensitive rashes), darkening of the skin, kidney damage, fluid retention, shock, inflammation of the heart, increase in symptoms of Lupus Erythematosus, swelling of the brain in infants, anemia and other blood disorders, darkening of teeth in children when taken by women in the last months of pregnancy or by children up to 8 years of age.

Warnings: Kidney disease can lead to excessive build-up in the system. Exaggerated skin irritation or sunburn occurs commonly with some tetracyclines. Avoid alcohol if patient has a history of liver disease. Causes birth defects in animals — avoid during first three months of pregnancy. Known to be present in mothers' milk — avoid drug or avoid nursing.

Possible Interactions: May interfere with the action of penicillin. Antacids, calcium supplements, epsom salts, sodium bicarbonate, or iron tonics may reduce absorption of this medication. Dairy products or vitamins containing iron should not be taken within 2-3 hours of the time tetracyclines are taken, since they may interfere with its action or absorption.

Theo-Dur® *(Key)*
See: Xanthine Class

Theolair™ *(Riker)*
See: Xanthine Class

Theophylline
See: Xanthine Class

Theragran Hematinic® *(Squibb)*

Category Of Drug: Vitamin/Mineral Supplement

Ingredients: Vitamin A + Vitamin D + Thiamine +

Riboflavin + Pyridoxine + Niacin + Calcium + Vitamin E +
Copper + Magnesium + Iron + Vitamin B12 + Vitamin C +
Folic Acid

Intended Effects: To treat many forms of iron-deficiency
anemia, particularly those associated with nutritional deficiency states, or when nutritional requirements are high.

Side Effects: Allergic reactions, skin rashes, stomach
disturbances, vomiting, nausea, diarrhea, constipation,
flushing and feeling of warmth.

Warnings: Should be used with caution by people with
gastritis, peptic ulcer, or asthma. Not for people with excessive deposits of iron in body tissues. Possibility of pernicious anemia should be excluded before treatment with this
drug. Contains tartrazine which may cause allergic reactions
(including bronchial asthma), most often in people who are
also allergic to aspirin.

Possible Interactions: Tetracyclines should not be taken
within two hours of taking this supplement since the iron in
it will interfere with the absorption of tetracycline. Mineral
oil and bile-acid products such as cholestyramine and colestipol decrease the absorption of some vitamins. Certain ingredients in this vitamin/mineral supplement may decrease the
effects of levodopa and anticlotting drugs. Neomycin, colchicine, colestipol, phenytoin, methotrexate, pyrimethamine,
hydralazine, penicillamine, isoniazid and cycloserine may
decrease the effects of individual ingredients in Theragran
Hematinic®.

Thiazide Diuretic Class

Generic / Brand Names:
Chlorothiazide/Diuril®
Chlorthalidone/Hygroton®
Hydrochlorothiazide/Esidrix®, HydroDIURIL®
Methyclothiazide/Enduron®
Metolazone/Diulo®, Zaroxolyn®

Category Of Drug: Blood-Pressure Reducer, Diuretic

Intended Effects: To reduce high blood pressure, to eliminate excess fluid from the body.

Side Effects: Loss of appetite, nausea, vomiting, cramping, diarrhea, constipation, jaundice, inflammation of the pancreas, dizziness, loss of balance, tingling sensations, headache, anemia and other blood disorders, bleeding under the skin, sensitivity to light, rashes, inflammation of blood vessels in the skin, fever, difficult breathing, congestion in the lungs, shock, high blood sugar, uremic poisoning, muscle spasms, weakness, restlessness, blurred vision.

Warnings: Should be used with caution by people with poor kidney function or progressive liver disease. Sensitivity reactions are more likely to occur in people with allergies or bronchial asthma. Can cause severe sunburn. May cause birth defects — avoid during pregnancy. Known to be present in mothers' milk — avoid drug or avoid nursing.

Possible Interactions: Thiazides may add to the action of other blood-pressure reducers. Insulin requirements may need to be adjusted. Potassium supplements or diets rich in citrus fruit or other sources of potassium may be recommended for those taking thiazide diuretics which lead to potassium loss. Potassium sparing drugs like spironolactone, triamterene or amiloride make potassium supplementation unnecessary and possibly harmful. Interacts with digitalis and related drugs, adrenocorticoids, tricyclic antidepressants. Pain relievers and barbiturates may cause increased effects. To avoid poisonous levels, do not take lithium.

Thioridazine
See: Phenothiazine Class

Thiothixene

Brand Name: Navane®

Category Of Drug: Tranquilizer

Intended Effects: To treat psychotic disorders.

Side Effects: Rapid heartbeat, lightheadedness, low blood pressure, drowsiness, restlessness, agitation, insomnia, rash, itching, hives, exaggerated sunburn, dry mouth, blurred vision, nasal congestion, constipation, increased sweating, increased salivation, changes in appetite, nausea, vomiting, weakness or fatigue. With long term use: (especially with high doses or in the elderly) involuntary movements of the tongue, mouth, jaw or face. Infrequent: seizures.

Warnings: Not for children under the age of 12, those with serious blood disorders or Parkinson's disease. Should be used with caution by people with glaucoma, epilepsy, heart disease, poor kidney or liver function, high blood pressure or people who drink alcoholic beverages regularly. Drive and operate machinery with caution.

Possible Interactions: Sedation may increase when taken with: tranquilizers, antihistamines, antidepressants, sedatives, sleep inducers, alcohol and narcotics. Brain wave patterns may be altered if this drug is taken with anticonvulsant drugs. This drug may lead to lower blood pressure in people taking blood-pressure reducers. May interact with many over-the-counter medications for coughs, colds or allergies.

Thorazine® (*Smith Kline & French*)
  See: Phenothiazine Class

Thyroglobulin
  See: Thyroid Hormone Class

Thyroxine
  See: Thyroid Hormone Class

Thyroid Hormone Class

Generic / Brand Names:
  Levothyroxine/ Synthroid®
  Liothyronine/ Cytomel®
  Liotrix/ Euthroid®, Thyrolar®
  Thyroglobulin/ Proloid®
  Thyroxine/ Levothroid®

Category Of Drug: Thyroid Hormone

Intended Effects: To combat low levels of thyroid hormone with associated symptoms such as depression, mental apathy, drowsiness, sensitivity to cold, constipation; to reduce the size of goiters.

Side Effects: No side effects should be present if replacement therapy brings thyroid levels up to the normal range. If dosage is too high, side effects may include nervousness, tremor in the hands, weakness, sensitivity to heat, reduced sweating, overactivity, weight loss, pounding heartbeat, bulging eyeballs, headache, nausea, abdominal pain, diarrhea, high blood pressure, and heart failure.

Warnings: Be alert for side effects which are signs that dosage should be reduced. After a few weeks, mild side effects may disappear as the body compensates by reducing its production of thyroid hormones. Should not be used to treat obesity except when medical studies show there is thyroid deficiency. Should be used with caution by diabetics, people recovering from recent heart attacks, people taking anticlotting drugs, people with heart disease, Addison's disease, or high blood pressure.

Possible Interactions: May increase the effects of anticlotting drugs, digitalis preparations, certain stimulants, and tricyclic antidepressants. May decrease the effects of barbiturates. Aspirin and phenytoin may increase the effects of thyroid. Dosages may need to be adjusted if antidiabetic drugs or adrenocorticoid drugs are taken with thyroid hormones.

Thyrolar® (*Usv*)
  See: Thyroid Hormone Class

Tigan® (*Beecham*)

See: Trimethobenzamide

Timolol
See: Beta-Adrenergic Blocking Agent Class
See: Timoptic®

Timoptic® *(Merck Sharp & Dohme)*

Category Of Drug: Antiglaucoma

Ingredients: Timolol

Intended Effects: To reduce pressure within the eye, especially in patients with glaucoma, by application directly to the eye in the form of drops.

Side Effects: Irritation of the eye and eyelids, rashes, hives, visual disturbances, swelling of tissue in the vicinity of the eye, potentially fatal breathing difficulties — especially in asthmatics, hypoglycemic reaction (see insulin for description).

Warnings: Present in mothers' milk. Avoid drug or avoid nursing.

Note: See Beta-Adrenergic Blocking Agent Class for other possible side effects, warnings and interactions. These should be reduced since the amount of the drug entering the body's system from the eye is less than that which would be present in oral or other forms of administration.

Tobrex® Ophthalmic *(Alcon)*

Category Of Drug: Antibiotic

Ingredients:
  <u>Ophthalmic Ointment</u> -- Tobramycin + Mineral Oil + Petrolatum Base + Chlorobutanol
  <u>Ophthalmic Solution</u> -- Tobramycin + Boric Acid + Sodium Sulfate + Sodium Chloride + Tyloxapol + Sodium Hydroxide + / or Sulfuric Acid + Purified Water + Benzalkonium Chloride

Intended Effects: To treat external eye infections.

Side Effects: Lid itching, swelling of the eye lids, swelling of the mucous membrane that covers the front of the eye, burning, stinging.

Warnings: Prolonged use of topical antibiotics may cause fungus infections. Ointments for the eye may hinder corneal healing. May be present in mothers' milk -- avoid drug or avoid nursing.

Possible Interactions: Serum concentration levels should be closely monitored if systemic aminoglycoside antibiotics are taken with Tobrex®.

Tocainide

Brand Name: Tonocard®

Category Of Drug: Heart-Rhythm Regulator

Intended Effects: To regulate heart rhythm.

Side Effects: Lightheadedness, dizziness, nausea,

numbness, tingling sensations, tremors, loss of balance, giddiness, quivering, confusion, disorientation, hallucinations, restlessness, shakiness, nervousness, incoordination, unsteadiness, difficulty in walking, anxiety, loss of appetite, sweating, clamminess, cold sweat, headache, low blood pressure, tiredness, drowsiness, sleepiness, chest pain, awareness of heartbeat, slow heartbeat, ringing in the ears, loss of hearing, hot or cold feelings, skin rash, diarrhea, loose stools, arthritis. Infrequent side effects: coma, convulsions, seizures, depression, altered taste, altered smell, difficulty in concentrating, loss of memory, nightmares, thirst, weakness, myasthenia gravis, stomach pain, constipation, difficult breathing, irregular heartbeat, blood disorders, anemia, dry mouth, earache, water retention, fever, hiccups, itching, leg cramps, "unwell" feeling, metallic taste, muscle twitching, neck pain, flushed face, loss of color, pressure on shoulder, yawning.

Warnings: Not for use in people allergic to anesthetics of the "amide" type, or in people with heart blocks. Any bruising, bleeding, fever, sore throat, cough, wheezing, difficult breathing or chills should be reported to the doctor immediately. Regular blood counts are recommended. Should be used with caution by people with known heart failure, a weak heart, severe liver or kidney disease, or a low potassium level. Taking tocainide with meals may help to lessen side effects.

Possible Interactions: None known.

Tofranil® (*Geigy*)
See: Tricyclic Antidepressant Class

Tolazamide
See: Antidiabetic Class

Tolbutamide
See: Antidiabetic Class

Tolectin® (*McNeil*)
See: Tolmetin

Tolinase® (*Upjohn*)
See: Antidiabetic Class

Tolmetin

Brand Name: Tolectin®

Category Of Drug: Anti-inflammatory, Pain Reliever

Intended Effects: To relieve inflammation and pain cause by osteoarthritis, rheumatoid arthritis, and juvenile rheumatoid arthritis.

Side Effects: Most frequent (7%-15%): nausea, upset stomach, headache, swelling and fluid retention. Frequent (1%-7%): passing gas, diarrhea, constipation, vomiting, stomach inflammation, peptic ulcer, weakness, chest pain, shock, high blood pressure, dizziness, nervousness, drowsiness, insomnia, depression, itching, skin rash, ringing in the ears. Rare (less than 1%): blood disorders and bleeding from the stomach without the presence of peptic ulcers.

Warnings: Long term use may contribute to cataract formation, although this has not been observed in humans; slight changes in the eye lens have been observed in animal studies. Should be used with caution by people with history of peptic ulcer, heart disease, poor kidney or liver function, or those taking anticlotting drugs. Prolongs bleeding time. Not for people who are allergic to aspirin or those with bleeding disorders or active stomach ulcer.

Possible Interactions: May increase the effects of anticlotting drugs. Avoid aspirin and aspirin-containing drugs, which may decrease the effects of this drug. May cause increased withdrawal effects from adrenocorticoids when such hormones are discontinued while taking tolmetin. Use with alcohol can cause increased chance of bleeding.

Tonocard® (*Merck Sharp & Dohme*)
  See: Tocainide

Topicort® (*Hoechst-Roussel*)
  See: Adrenocorticoid Class-Topical

Tornalate® (*Winthrop-Breon*)
  See: Bitolterol Mesylate

Totacillin® (*Glaxo*)
  See: Penicillin Class

Trandate® (*Glaxo*)
  See: Labetalol

Transderm-Nitro® (*CIBA*)
  See: Nitroglycerin — Topical

Tranxene® (*Abbott*)
  See: Benzodiazepine Class

Tranylcypromine
  See: Monoamine Oxidase Inhibitor Class

Trazodone

Brand Name: Desyrel®

Category Of Drug: Antidepressant

Intended Effects: To treat depression.

Side Effects: Nausea, vomiting, drowsiness, dizziness, dry mouth, blurred vision, sudden stopping of breathing, double vision, water retention, hallucinations, hemolytic anemia, tingling sensations, persistent erection of the penis, rash, weakness, changes in blood pressure, awareness of heartbeat, fainting, slow, rapid or irregular heartbeat, heart attack, shortness of breath, anger, hostility, nightmares, vivid dreams, confusion, disorientation, lowered concentration, lightheadedness, excitement, tiredness, headache, inability to sleep, poor memory, nervousness, incoordination, ringing in the ears, tired or red eyes, stuffy nose, increased or decreased sex drive, impotence, missed periods, bad taste, constipation, muscle aches and pains, irregular urination, changes in appetite, sweating, clamminess, weight gain or loss.

Warnings: Should be used cautiously in patients with heart conditions. Take immediately after meals or a snack Alert doctor to signs of infections (sore throat or fever) that may indicate a low white blood cell count. Avoid electroshock treatments. Causes birth defects in animals — avoid during first three months of pregnancy. Known to be present in mothers' milk — avoid drug or avoid nursing.

Possible Interactions: May increase the effects of other antidepressants, digoxin, phenytoin, antihistamines, sedatives, sleep inducers, alcohol and narcotics. Use cautiously with MAO inhibitors as possible interactions are not known. Dosage of blood-pressure reducers may need to be adjusted. May decrease the effect of clonidine. May react with general anesthetics — should be discontinued before surgery.

Trental® (*Hoechst-Roussel*)
 See: Pentoxifylline

Tretinoin

Brand Name: Retin-A®

Category Of Drug: Anti-acne

Intended Effects: To treat acne.

Side Effects: Sun-sensitivity, redness, blistering, crusting or swelling of the skin. Temporary darkening or lightening of the skin at treated area, feeling of warmth, mild stinging. Peeling of skin may occur a few days after treatment.

Warnings: People using this drug should avoid or minimize exposure to the sun. Wind or cold may be irritating. Not for use near the eyes, mouth, angles of the nose, or mucous membranes. Should be used with extreme caution by people with eczema.

Possible Interactions: May interact with other topical acne preparations, especially those containing peeling agents such as sulfur, resorcinol, benzoyl peroxide or salicylic acid. Medicated or abrasive soaps and cleansers, cosmetics and soaps which cause drying, and products which contain high concentrations of astringents, spices, lime or alcohol may interact with tretinoin and cause irritation.

Triamcinolone

See: Adrenocorticoid Class - Systemic or Topical

Triamterene

Brand Name: Dyrenium®

Category Of Drug: Diuretic, Blood-Pressure Reducer

Intended Effects: To eliminate excessive fluid retention associated with congestive heart failure, cirrhosis of the liver, or several types of fluid retention, without loss of potassium from the body.

Side Effects: Nausea, vomiting, diarrhea, weakness, headache, dry mouth, excessive sunburn, allergic rash. Rare: bone marrow depression, anemia.

Warnings: Known to be present in mothers' milk — avoid drug or avoid nursing. Not for people with severe kidney or liver disease or impairment. Should be used with caution by people with diabetes, gout, those taking any form of digitalis, or those with history of kidney stone formation.

Possible Interactions: Do not use with other potassium-sparing drugs such as spironolactone or amiloride. May increase the effects of other high blood pressure drugs. May decrease the effects of anti-diabetic drugs and digitalis preparations. Do not take with potassium supplements.

Triavil® (*Merck Sharp & Dohme*)
   See: Phenothiazine Class
   See: Tricyclic Antidepressant Class

Triazolam

Brand Name: Halcion®

Category Of Drug: Sleeping Aid

Intended Effect: To induce sleep.

Side Effects: Drowsiness, dizziness, lightheadedness, headache, nervousness, incoordination, nausea, vomiting, excessive feeling of happiness, increased heart rate, tiredness, confusion, poor memory, cramps, pain, depression, visual disturbances, constipation, altered taste, diarrhea, dry mouth, inflammation of the skin, vivid dreams, nightmares, inability to sleep, tingling sensations, ringing in the ears, weakness, congestion, liver failure, irritability, loss of appetite, tiredness, slurred speech, itching, changes in sex drive, irregular menstruation, poor urinary control, stimulation, agitation, muscle spasms in the back, sleep disturbances, hallucinations.

Warnings: May be physically and psychologically habit-forming. Do not discontinue abruptly — gradual withdrawal is recommended after extensive use. Do not use in small children or in people sensitive to benzodiazepines. Causes severe birth defects — avoid during pregnancy. Should be avoided by women of childbearing potential if not using effective contraception. May be present in mothers' milk — avoid drug or avoid nursing. Use with caution in elderly or depressed people or those with poor kidney or liver function. Avoid alcohol. Because of sedation, drive or operate machinery with caution.

Possible Interactions: Sedation may increase when taken with: other sleep inducers, tranquilizers, antihistamines, antidepressants, sedatives, alcohol or narcotics.

Note: See Benzodiazepine Class

Tricyclic Antidepressant Class

Generic / Brand Names:
  Amitriptyline/Elavil®
  Desipramine/Norpramin®
  Doxepin/Adapin®,Sinequan®
  Imipramine/Tofranil®
  Maprotiline/Ludiomil®

Perphenazine + Amitriptyline/Triavil®

Category Of Drug: Antidepressant

Intended Effects: To treat depressive illnesses such as depressive neurosis, manic-depressive illness, depressed type, and to relieve anxiety associated with depression. To treat depressions associated with alcoholism.

Side Effects: Change in blood pressure, skipped or pounding heartbeat, heart attacks, congestive heart failure, stroke, hallucinations, delusions, anxiety, agitation, insomnia, manic behavior, tingling sensations, tremors, seizure, ringing in the ears, dryness of the mouth, blurred vision, constipation, urinary retention, skin rashes including light-sensitive skin rashes, fluid retention, depression, low bone marrow count, blood disorders, nausea, vomiting, diarrhea, cramps, enlargement of the breasts in males and females, discharge of fluid from the breasts in females, changed sex drive, impotence, swelling of the testicles, low or high blood sugar levels, jaundice, weight gain or loss, perspiration, flushing of the skin, frequent urination, drowsiness, dizziness, weakness, fatigue, headache, loss of balance.

Warnings: The therapeutic effects of antidepressants may not be evident for a few weeks, so do not discontinue their use because the desired effect is not achieved immediately. There are at least three major neuro-hormones which may be out of balance in cases of depression. Different antidepressants affect these neuro-hormones in different ways, so it may be necessary for physician to try different antidepressants and/or major tranquilizers before the desired effect is achieved. Exercise caution in cases of cardio-vascular disease, increased pressure within the eyes and in people who have a history of seizures. Avoid taking during the recovery period after a heart attack. Avoid alcohol.

314

Possible Interactions: Sedation may increase when taken with: tranquilizers, antihistamines, antidepressants, sedatives, sleep inducers, alcohol and narcotics. Convulsions may result when taken with MAO inhibitors. May increase the effects of levodopa. When taken with thyroid hormone or quinidine, may cause abnormalities in heartbeat. When taken with blood-pressure reducers, may reduce their effectiveness.

Tridesilon® (*Miles*)
  See: Adrenocorticoid Class-Topical

Trifluoperazine
  See: Phenothiazine Class

Trihexyphenidyl
  See: Antidyskinetic Class

Trilafon® (*Schering*)
  See: Phenothiazine Class

Trilisate® (*Purdue*)
  See: Salicylate Class

Trimeprazine

Brand Name: Temaril®

Category Of Drug: Anti-itching

Intended Effects: To relieve itching from hives, chicken pox, allergic dermatitis and other skin disorders.

Side Effects: Drowsiness, dry mouth, blurred vision, poor concentration, headache, ringing in the ears, incoordination, fatigue, euphoria, nervousness, insomnia, tremors, excitation, disturbing dreams, loss of appetite, nausea, vomiting, frequent urination, retention, thickening of bronchial secretions, tightness of the chest, wheezing, asthma, lightheadedness, faintness, dizziness, tiredness, diarrhea, constipation, dry mouth, increased appetite, weight gain, asthma. Rare: liver disease, poor vision, skin rash.

Warnings: Should be used with extreme caution in patients with asthma, narrow-angle glaucoma, enlarged prostate, peptic ulcer, bladder neck or duodenal obstruction. Should be used cautiously in people with chronic poor breathing (especially children), history of ulcers, poor liver function, or heart disease. Not for those with bone marrow depression, newborn or premature children, seriously ill children or children with history of Sudden Infant Death Syndrome in the family. Use caution when driving or operating machinery. May reduce mental alertness in children. Not for people who have shown sensitivity to phenothiazines.

Possible Interactions: Sedation may increase when taken with: tranquilizers, antihistamines, antidepressants, sedatives, sleep inducers, alcohol and narcotics. May block or reverse the effects of epinephrine.

Trimethobenzamide

316

Brand Name: Tigan®

Category Of Drug: Antivomiting

Intended Effects: To control nausea and vomiting.

Side Effects: Tremor, low blood pressure, blood disorders, blurred vision, coma, convulsions, depressed mood, diarrhea, disorientation, drowsiness, dizziness, headache, jaundice, muscle cramps, allergic skin reactions such as hives and rashes.

Warnings: The use of this drug to treat symptoms may mask the causes of nausea and vomiting. When given to combat viral illnesses, may produce disorders of the nervous system such as Reye's Syndrome, with symptoms such as high fever and lack of muscle control. May also cause symptoms which only mimic those of Reye's Syndrome with loss of muscle control. Drive and operate machinery with caution, because of possible drowsiness.

Possible Interactions: Should not be taken by people who are sensitive to benzocaine-related drugs, which are used in suppositories containing trimethobenzamide. Sedation may increase when taken with: tranquilizers, antihistamines, antidepressants, sedatives, sleep inducers, alcohol and narcotics.

Trimethoprim + Sulfamethoxazole
  See: Sulfonamide Class - Systemic or Topical

Trimox® *(Squibb)*
  See: Penicillin Class

Trinalin® (*Schering*)
See: Antihistamine Class

Trinsicon® (*Glaxo*)

Category Of Drug: Vitamin/Mineral Supplement

Ingredients: Special Liver-Stomach Concentrate + Cobalamin + Iron + Ascorbic Acid + Folic Acid

Intended Effects: To prevent or correct iron-deficiency anemia, pernicious anemia and other anemias.

Side Effects: Allergic sensitization has been reported following administration of folic acid. Can cause harmless gray to black discoloration of stools. Rare: diarrhea, constipation, or skin rash.

Warnings: Unneeded iron taken on a continuous basis may be hazardous. This drug should be taken only by people who actually are iron-deficient. Do not exceed dosage needed to correct the anemia. Not for people who have excessive deposits of iron in body tissues, those with hemolytic anemia or those with acute hepatitis. Should be used with caution by those with ulcerative colitis, inflammation of the small intestine, peptic ulcer, and those who abuse alcohol.

Possible Interactions: Decreases the effect of tetracyclines. Alcohol, antacids, eggs, tea or whole grain breads and cereals will decrease iron absorption, as will food or medications containing bicarbonates, carbonates, oxalates, or phosphates.

Tripelennamine
See: Antihistamine Class

Triphasil 21® (*Wyeth*)
See: Estrogen + Progestin Class

Tri-Vi-Flor® (*Mead Johnson*)

Category Of Drug: Vitamin/Mineral Supplement

Ingredients: Vitamins A + D + C + Fluoride

Intended Effects: To provide vitamin and fluoride supplementation during tooth development, to aid in preventing future tooth decay.

Side Effects: Rare: allergic rash.

Warnings: Do not exceed recommended dosage. Not for infants from birth to age 2 in areas where the drinking water contains 0.3ppm or more fluoride. Not for children ages 2-3 in areas where the drinking water contains more than 0.7ppm fluoride (ppm = parts per million).

Tussend® (*Merrell Dow*)

Category Of Drug: Anticough, Decongestant

Ingredients: Hydrocodone + Pseudoephedrine + Alcohol

Intended Effects: To relieve coughing and upper respiratory tract congestion in association with the common cold, flu, bronchitis and sinusitis.

Side Effects: Drowsiness, stomach upset, nausea, constipation, pounding or irregular heartbeat, headache, dizziness, anxiety, tenseness, restlessness, tremor, weakness, respiratory difficulty, insomnia, hallucinations, convulsions, or central nervous system depression.

Warnings: Not for people with severe high blood pressure, severe coronary artery disease, sensitivity to decongestants or bronchial-tube relaxers. Extreme caution should be used by people with breathing disorders. Caution should be exercised by people with high blood pressure, diabetes, coronary heart disease, overactive thyroid, increased pressure within the eye or enlarged prostate. Drive and operate machinery with caution. Do not exceed recommended dosage. Very high doses over a long period of time may produce psychological and physical dependence.

Possible Interactions: Sedation may increase when taken with: tranquilizers, antihistamines, antidepressants, sedatives, sleep inducers, alcohol and narcotics. Do not use with MAO inhibitors.

Tussend® Expectorant *(Merrell Dow)*

Category Of Drug: Anticough, Decongestant, Phlegm Loosener

Ingredients: Hydrocodone + Pseudoephedrine + Guaifenesin + Alcohol

Intended Effects: To relieve coughing and upper respiratory tract congestion in the common cold, flu, bronchitis and sinusitis; to promote productive coughing by loosening phlegm.

Note: See Tussend
See Guaifenesin

Tussionex® *(Pennwalt)*

Category Of Drug: Anticough

Ingredients: Hydrocodone + Phenyltoloxamine

Intended Effects: To reduce persistent coughing.

Side Effects: Rare: constipation, nausea, facial itching, drowsiness. With overdose: convulsions, low breathing rates and loss of consciousness.

Warnings: Causes birth defects in animals — avoid during first three months of pregnancy. May be present in mothers' milk — avoid drug or avoid nursing. Large doses of this drug over an extended period of time may produce psychological and physical dependence. Young children are susceptible to suppression of breathing; estimation of dosage relative to the age and weight of the child is of great importance. Drive and operate machinery with caution.

Possible Interactions: Sedation may increase when taken with tranquilizers, antihistamines, antidepressants, sedatives, sleep inducers, alcohol and narcotics.

Tussi-Organidin® *(Wallace)*

Category Of Drug: Anticough, Phlegm Loosener, Antihistamine

Ingredients: Organidin® + Codeine + Alcohol

Intended Effects: To prevent excessive coughing, to aid in productive coughing by loosening phlegm.

Side Effects: May produce excitation, especially in children. May cause a flare-up of adolescent acne. Most reported side effects with this combination of drugs have been rare. They are, by ingredient: (Organidin®) stomach irritation, rash, hypersensitivity, thyroid gland enlargement; (codeine) nausea, vomiting, constipation, drowsiness, dizziness.

Warnings: Children with cystic fibrosis appear to have an exaggerated susceptibility to goiter-producing effects. Not for people with marked sensitivity to iodine compounds or newborn infants. Discontinue use if rash or other evidence of sensitivity appears. Use with caution or avoid in people with history or evidence of thyroid disease. Drive and operate machinery with caution.

Possible Interactions: May increase the thyroid hormone lowering effects of lithium and other antithyroid drugs. MAO inhibitors may prolong the drying effects. Sedation may increase when taken with: tranquilizers, antihistamines, antidepressants, sedatives, sleep inducers, alcohol and narcotics.

Note: See Codeine

Tuss-Ornade® (*Smith Kline & French*)

Category Of Drug: Anticough, Bronchial-Tube Relaxer, Decongestant

Ingredients: Caramiphen Edisylate + Phenylpropanolamine

Intended Effects: To relieve coughs and nasal congestion associated with common colds.

Side Effects: Dryness of nose, throat or mouth, nervousness, insomnia, nausea, vomiting, stomach distress, diarrhea, dizziness, weakness, tightness of chest, pain of angina pectoris, abdominal pain, irritability, pounding heartbeat, headache, tremor, urinary problems, blood pressure disorders, loss of appetite, constipation, visual disturbances, acne, drowsiness, incoordinated movements.

Warnings: May interfere with milk flow in nursing mothers. Use cautiously in people with heart or blood vessel disease, glaucoma, enlargement of the prostate and over-active thyroid. Allergic reactions may occur in people who are sensitive to yellow dye #5 or aspirin. Do not use in cases of severe high blood pressure, asthma, peptic ulcer, intestinal or bladder obstructions. Do not use Tuss-Ornade® liquid in children under 15 pounds or in children less than 6 months of age. Do not use the timed-release Tuss-Ornade® Spansules® in children under 12, because they contain higher doses than are recommended for children.

Possible Interactions: Do not take with MAO inhibitors. Patients taking this drug should not take other products containing phenylpropanolamine or amphetamines at the same time. Sedation may increase when taken with: tranquilizers, antihistamines, antidepressants, sedatives, sleep inducers, alcohol and narcotics.

Tylenol® (*McNeil*)
See: Acetaminophen

Note: No Rx prescription required

Tylenol® + Codeine (*McNeil*)
See: Acetaminophen
See: Codeine

Note: Numbers 1,2,3 or 4 indicate increasing amounts of codeine.

Tylox® (*McNeil*)
See: Acetaminophen
See: Oxycodone

Urecholine® (*Merck Sharp & Dohme*)
See: Bethanechol

Urised® (*Webcon*)

Category Of Drug: Anti-infective

Ingredients: Methenamine + Phenyl Salicylate + Methylene Blue + Benzoic Acid + Atropine + Hyoscyamine

Intended Effects: To suppress and control long term or recurring urinary tract (kidney and bladder) infections.

Side Effects: Dryness of mouth, flushing, difficult urination, rapid pulse, dizziness, blurred vision, blue to blue-green urine, discolored stools. With large doses over an extended period of time: bladder and stomach irritation, painful and frequent urination, albumin in the urine.

Warnings: Not for patients with glaucoma, urinary bladder neck obstruction, stomach or duodenal obstruction, or heart spasms. Use with great caution in those with severe kidney or liver disease, in people with reactions to atropine-like compounds, and people suffering from heart disease.

Possible Interactions: Use of this drug with sulfonamides is not recommended since formation of crystals in the kidneys and kidney destruction may result. Drugs or foods which produce an alkaline urine should be restricted.

Valisone® (*Schering*)
   See: Adrenocorticoid Class (Topical)   *Page 38*

Valium® (*Roche*)
   See: Benzodiazepine Class

Valproic Acid

Brand Name: Depakene®

Category Of Drug: Anticonvulsant

Intended Effects: To treat seizures which involve a brief loss of consciousness, including petit mal seizures; to help in the treatment of other seizures.

Side Effects: Nausea, vomiting, indigestion, diarrhea, abdominal cramps, constipation, emotional upset, depression, aggression, hyperactivity, loss of appetite with weight loss, increased appetite with weight gain, headache, tremors, dizziness, incoordination, skin rash, weakness, and bruising.

Warnings: Use with extreme caution in cases of kidney or liver disease. Do not discontinue this drug abruptly since seizures may occur. Drive and use hazardous machinery with caution. Affects bleeding time — treatment may be changed before surgery.

Possible Interactions: May cause prolonged bleeding time if taken with aspirin or anticlotting drugs, especially warfarin. May cause petit mal seizures if taken with clonazepam. Dosage of phenytoin, barbiturates or primidone may need to be adjusted if taken with this drug. Sedation may increase when taken with: tranquilizers, antihistamines, antidepressants, sedatives, sleep inducers, alcohol and narcotics. Naloxone should be used with caution.

Vanceril® (*Schering*)
  See: Beclomethasone

Vasocidin® Ophthalmic Solution
                              (*CooperVision*)
Category Of Drug: Anti-infective

Ingredients: Sulfacetamide + Prednisolone + Phenyleph-rine

Intended Effects: To treat bacterial infections of the eye.

Side Effects: Itching, swelling, redness, or other signs of irritation not present before use of this drug. Prolonged use may result in glaucoma, optic nerve damage, visual defects, formation of cataracts, or eye infections. May lead to perfo-ration of the cornea in diseases causing thinning of the cor-nea.

Warnings: Not for people with herpes simplex, keratitis, cowpox, chickenpox, viral diseases of the eye and eyelids, tuberculosis and fungus diseases of the eye, narrow angle glaucoma, or in people who react to adrenocorticoids. Do not use this medicine if it turns dark brown.

Possible Interactions: Local anesthetics related to p-aminobenzoic acid may decrease the action of sulfonamides. Do not use with solutions containing silver preparations.

Vasocon-A® Ophthalmic (*CooperVision*)

Category Of Drug: Blood-Vessel Narrower

Ingredients: Naphazoline + Antazoline (in an ophthalmic solution)

Intended Effects: To relieve congestion, minor irritation and itching of the eye caused by pollen-related allergies, in-flammatory or infectious conditions.

Side Effects: Pupil dilation, increase in pressure within the eye. Rare: high blood pressure, heart irregularities, excess sugar in the blood, drowsiness. Coma may occur in young children.

Warnings: Should be used with caution by people with high blood pressure, heart irregularities and diabetes. Excessive sedation may result if this drug is used in infants and children — use is not recommended. Not for people with narrow-angle glaucoma.

Possible Interactions: Use with MAO inhibitors may result in severe rise in blood pressure.

Vasodilan® (*Mead Johnson*)
See: Isoxsuprine

Vasotec® (*Merck Sharp & Dohme*)
See: Angiotensin Converting Enzyme Inhibitor Class

V-Cillin K® (*Lilly*)
See: Penicillin Class

Velosef® (*Squibb*)
See: Cephalosporin Class

Ventolin® (*Glaxo*)
See: Albuterol

Verapamil
See: Calcium Channel Inhibitors

Vermox® (*Janssen*)
See: Mebendazole

Vibramycin® (*Pfizer*)
See: Tetracycline Class

Vibra-Tabs® (*Pfizer*)
See: Tetracycline Class

Vicodin® (*Knoll*)

Category Of Drug: Pain Reliever, Fever Reducer

Ingredients: Hydrocodone + Acetaminophen

Intended Effects: To relieve moderate to moderately severe pain.

Side Effects: Sedation, drowsiness, lethargy, poor physical and mental performance, anxiety, fear, dizziness, mood changes, unhappy feelings, nausea, vomiting, constipation, urinary retention, urethral spasm interfering with urination, breathing problems.

Warnings: Drug dependence may develop. Should be used with caution after surgery in the elderly or infirm, in those with very poor kidney or liver function, lung disease, underactive thyroid, Addison's disease, enlarged prostate or urethral constriction. Drive and operate machinery with caution. Use with extreme caution in cases of head injury, increased pressure within the skull, or acute abdominal conditions. Causes birth defects in animals — avoid during first three months of pregnancy.

Possible Interactions: Sedation may increase when taken with: tranquilizers, antihistamines, antidepressants, sedatives, sleep inducers, alcohol and narcotics. When used with MAO inhibitors or tricyclic antidepressants may increase the effects of these drugs. Use of nervous-system regulators with this drug may cause normal movement within the intestines to stop.

Vioform®-Hydrocortisone (*CIBA*)

Category Of Drug: Adrenal Hormone, Antifungus, Anti-infective, Anti-inflammatory

Ingredients: Iodochlorhydroxyquin + Hydrocortisone

Intended Effects: To reduce allergic reactions associated with many skin diseases; to combat infections by certain susceptible micro-organisms such as fungi and cocci.

Side Effects: Rash, burning, itching, irritation, skin dryness, skin eruptions, loss of pigmentation from the skin, infection by nonsusceptible organisms.

Warnings: Discontinue treatment if irritations or allergic reactions occur. Other adrenocorticoid side effects, warnings and interactions should be absent or mild if use is limited to small areas in older children and adults. If used in young children, or over large areas, or if used under other dressings, enough may be absorbed into the body's system to interfere with the functioning of the adrenal glands. Not for use in eyes. May stain skin and fabrics. Not for people with eye injuries, tuberculosis of the skin, or most viral skin problems. Continue use for full duration of treatment.

Note: See Adrenocorticoid Class-Systemic or Topical

Visken® (*Sandoz*)
See. Beta-Adrenergic Blocking Agent Class

Vistaril® (*Pfizer*)
See: Hydroxyzine Class

Vitamin C
See: Ascorbic Acid

VoSol® HC Otic Solution (*Wallace*)

Category Of Drug: Antifungus, Anti-inflammatory, Anti-itching, Anti-infective

Ingredients: Hydrocortisone + Acetic Acid Otic Solution

Intended Effects: To treat superficial, inflamed infections of the outer ear canal.

Side Effects: Stinging, burning, itching in the ear.

Warnings: Not for people with perforated eardrum, cow-pox or chicken-pox. Causes birth defects in animals — avoid during first three months of pregnancy. Known to be present in mothers' milk — avoid drug or avoid nursing. Systemic side effects may occur with extensive use of steroids.

Note: See Adrenocorticoid Class-Systemic or Topical

Warfarin

Brand Name: Coumadin®

Category Of Drug: Anticlotting

Intended Effects: To treat victims of stroke, heart attack, or blood clots by reducing the ability of blood to clot.

Side Effects: Fever, nausea, diarrhea, stomach cramps, skin rash, hives. Consult physician if unusual bleeding occurs.

Warnings: Dosage should be carefully watched. Do not take additional drugs without physician's guidance. Causes birth defects in animals — avoid during pregnancy. Known to be present in mothers' milk — avoid drug or avoid nursing. People with history of abnormal bleeding, ulcerative colitis or active peptic ulcer should avoid this drug. Discontinue this medication gradually.

Possible Interactions: May increase the effects of some antidiabetics, insulin and phenytoin. Avoid anticlotting drugs with streptokinase or urokinase. People taking any additional medications should be carefully watched by physician. This drug may increase the effect of any other drug with anticlotting properties. The following drugs cause increased effects: alcohol, allopurinol, aspirin, anabolic steroids, antibiotics, bromelains, chloral hydrate, chlorpropamide, chymotrypsin, cimetidine, cinchophen, clofibrate, dextran, dextrothyroxine, diazoxide, dietary deficiencies, diuretics, disulfiram, drugs affecting blood elements, ethacrynic acid, fenoprofen, glucagon, hepatotoxic drugs, ibuprofen, indomethacin, inhalation anesthetics, mefenamic acid, methyldopa, methylphenidate, metronidazole, MAO inhibitors, nalidixic acid, naproxen, oxolinic acid, oxyphenbutazone, pyrazolones, phenylbutazone, phenyramidol, phenytoin, prolonged narcotics, quinidine, quinine, salicylates, sulfinpyrazone, sulfonamides, sulindac, thyroid drugs, tolbutamide, triclofos sodium, trimethoprim/sulfamethoxazole. The following drugs may cause decreased effects: adrenal hormones, alcohol, antacids, antihistamines, barbiturates, carbamazepine, chloral hydrate, chlordiazepoxide, cholestyramine, diet high in vitamin K, diuretics, glutethimide, griseofulvin, haloperidol, meprobamate, oral contraceptives, paraldehyde, primidone, rifampin, vitamin C.

Westcort® (*Westwood*)
See: Adrenocorticoids Class-Topical

Wyanoids® HC (*Wyeth*)

Category Of Drug: Anti-inflammatory, Rectal Suppositories

Ingredients: Hydrocortisone + Belladonna + Ephedrine + Boric Acid + Bismuth + Peruvian Balsam

Intended Effects: To treat the rectal inflammation which usually accompanies ulcerative colitis; to treat hemorrhoids.

Side Effects: Infection at treatment site, dry mouth, rapidpulse, blurred vision, dizziness.

Warnings: Should not be used by people with glaucoma or narrowing of the stomach outlet. Use with caution in people with enlarged prostate, urinary retention, the elderly, and children under the age of six. Should be discontinued if eye pain occurs, since this may indicate undiagnosed glaucoma. Frequent or prolonged use should be avoided.

Note: See Adrenocorticoid Class-Systemic

Wygesic® (*Wyeth*)

Category Of Drug: Pain Reliever, Narcotic

Ingredients: Propoxyphene + Acetaminophen

Intended Effects: To relieve mild to moderate pain occurring alone or with fever.

Side Effects: Infrequent (less than 1%): dizziness, sedation, nausea (lying down may relieve feeling of nausea.), vomiting. Rare: constipation, abdominal pain, skin rashes, light-headedness, headache, weakness, mood changes, minor visual disturbances, liver dysfunction.

Warnings: Not for people who are addiction-prone, or suicidal. Should be used with extreme caution by people who use alcohol to excess, or by those who take tranquilizers or antidepressants. Large doses over an extended period of time can produce physical and psychological dependence. Drive and operate machinery with caution. Not recommended for children under the age of 12. Known to be present in mothers' milk — avoid drug or avoid nursing.

Possible Interactions: Sedation may increase when taken with: tranquilizers, antihistamines, antidepressants, sedatives, sleep inducers, alcohol and narcotics.

Wymox® (*Wyeth*)
See: Penicillin Class

Xanax® (*Upjohn*)
See: Benzodiazepine Class

Xanthine Class

Generic / Brand Names:
Aminophylline
Dyphylline/Lufyllin®
Oxtriphylline/Choledyl®
Theophylline/Elixophyllin®, Slo-Phyllin®, Theo-Dur®, Theolair®

Category Of Drug: Bronchial-Tube Relaxer

Intended Effects: To treat bronchial asthma, bronchitis, emphysema and other disorders involving the lungs.

Side Effects: Nausea, vomiting, stomach pain, nervousness, rapid breathing, loss of appetite, headaches, irritability, restlessness, insomnia, muscle twitching, convulsions, heartbeat disorders, low blood pressure, shock, high blood sugar, interference with kidney function.

Warnings: Should be used cautiously in patients with heart disease, peptic ulcer, high blood pressure, over-active thyroid, injury to the heart or lungs, liver disease, the elderly, infants, and by people with congestive heart disease. Tablets should not be chewed or crushed.

Possible Interactions: May increase diuretic effects when taken with diuretics. May interfere with the rhythm of the heart when taken with rauwolfia drugs. May increase the elimination of lithium. May act against the effects of beta-blocking high blood pressure medicines. Barbecued foods and high protein diets reduce the effects of theophylline. May decrease the effectiveness of hexamethonium. Erythromycin may increase the levels of xanthines in the blood. Xanthines may increase the action of chlordiazepoxide. Concurrent use of other xanthine containing drugs may cause serious side effects. Smokers may need larger doses of xanthine drugs.

Xylocaine® Viscous (*Astra*)

Category Of Drug: Local Anesthetic (topical)

Ingredients: Lidocaine

Intended Effects: To treat irritated or inflamed mucous membranes of the mouth and throat.

Side Effects: Systemic side effects are very rare with this drug. They may include: nervousness, dizziness, blurred vision, tremors, drowsiness, convulsions, lowered blood tissues.

Uric Acid Reducer — To decrease levels of uric acid in the blood and thus combat gout and other problems related to excessive uric acid levels.

Uticaria — A splotchy rash usually called hives.

Vaccine — A solution of altered bacteria or virus which, when injected, provides immunity to the original disease-causing bacteria or virus without serious harmful effects.

Vasoconstrictor — See: Blood Vessel Narrower

Vasodilator — See: Blood Vessel Enlarger.

Vertigo — Loss of balance.

Vitamin — Organic chemical which is essential for normal chemical reactions in the body.

Vitamin Supplement — Extra vitamins used to supplement or add to those found in the diet.

Vitamin/Mineral Supplement — Extra vitamins and minerals used to add to those found in the diet.

Water Pills — See: Diuretic.

358

Lederle Laboratories
Div. of American Cyanamid Company
One Cyanamid Plaza
Wayne, NJ 07470

Lilly (Eli) and Company
Medical Department
307 E. McCarty Street
Indianapolis, IN 46285

Marion Laboratories, Inc.
Pharmaceutical Division
Marion Industrial Park
10236 Bunker Ridge Road
Kansas City, MO 64137

McNeil Pharmaceutical
McNeilab, Inc.
Spring House, PA 19477

**Mead Johnson
Pharmaceutical Division**
Mead Johnson & Company
2404 W. Pennsylvania Street
Evansville, IN 47721

Merck Sharpe & Dohme
Div. of Merck & Co., Inc.
West Point, PA 19486

**Merrell Dow Pharmaceuticals,
Inc.**
Subsidiary of The Dow Chemical
Company
Cincinnati, OH 45214

Miles Pharmaceuticals
Div. of Miles Laboratories, Inc.
400 Morgan Lane
West Haven, CT 06516

**Norwich Eaton
Pharmaceuticals, Inc.**
Medical Department
Norwich, NY 13815

Ortho Pharmaceutical Corp.
Medical Research Department
Raritan, NJ 08869

Parke-Davis
Div. Warner-Lambert, Inc.
201 Tabor Road
Morris Plains, NJ 07950

**Pennwalt Pharmaceutical
Division**
Pennwalt Corporation
755 Jefferson Road
Rochester, NY 14623

Pfipharmecs Division
Pfizer Inc.
235 E. 42nd Street
New York, NY 10017

Pfizer Laboratories Division
Pfizer, Inc.
235 E 42nd Street
New York, NY 10017

Pharmacia Laboratories
Div. of Pharmacia, Inc.
800 Centennial Avenue
Piscataway, NJ 08854

The Purdue Frederick Company
100 Connecticut Avenue
Norwalk, CT 06854

Reed & Carnrick
1 New England Avenue
Piscataway, NJ 08854

Riker Laboratories, Inc.
Subsidiary of 3M Company
19901 Nordhoff Street
Northridge, CA 91324

"Do You Know These Natural Health Secrets and Cures?"

(By Frank K. Wood)

FC&A, a nearby Peachtree City, Georgia, health publisher announced today the release of a new, $9.95 book for the general public, *"Encyclopedia of Natural Health Secrets and Cures"*.

LOOK AT THESE LIFE AND HEALTH SAVING SECRETS REVEALED IN THIS NEW BOOK

"We're so positive that one of our health tips or cures will work for you that we'll send you a free gift just for trying them."

- Senility doesn't have to happen. This pleasant remedy does wonders to help people think and feel young.
- Cancer from your electric wires? Don't laugh.
- Alzheimer's Disease. Something to avoid that may cause it.
- Sexual activity and memory loss. What's the connection?
- Stop dieting! Easy way to lose weight.
- Avoid arthritis symptoms. Do this.
- Feel warm in the winter. Try this.
- Zap a cold. Suck on this (it's not what you think).
- Hair loss in women. How you can stop it.
- Wrinkle reduction: tips from an expert.
- Cancer from your basement? Check this.
- Low I.Q.? It may be the way you sleep.
- A dramatic new way to avoid allergies.
- How tomatoes can help prevent this bowel problem.
- Asthma? Stop doing this and avoid attacks.
- Incontinence: this helps.
- This mineral lowers blood pressure.
- Bronchitis: an easily prevented cause.
- The water you drink may keep you from getting cancer.
- This kind of apple a day won't keep the doctor away.
- Women: how to help avoid breast cancer.
- A laxative that causes cancer.
- Watch the weather. It can cause a heart attack.
- Women who don't take this have three times as many heart attacks.
- Too much of this vitamin can kill you.
- How love helps your health.
- A common beverage that helps constipation.
- Dandruff: get rid of it this natural way.
- Keep your teeth. This works wonders.
- Don't grit your teeth. Take this.
- Relief for denture wearers.
- Feel happy, not sad, this way.
- Depression: a nutritional deficiency that can cause it.
- How plants can help this mysterious ailment.
- Diarrhea? Drink this.
- This helps a nagging female problem.
- Epilepsy? Here's help.
- Help for eye problems.
- Help non-cancerous breast lumps go away.
- Oh, my aching feet! Here's blessed relief.
- Gas? Little-known causes.
- Sore gums? Rub this on them.
- This hiccup cure also works well for headaches.
- Help for hearing problems.
- The protective power of prayer.
- Heart surgery? An alternative.
- A simple trick that helps increase fertility.
- Headaches from your cups and saucers?
- Leg cramp prevention.
- Help for women past menopause.
- Pain in the joints. This can help.
- How to get pregnant.
- Premenstrual Syndrome. Here's relief.
- Heartbreak of psoriasis? A new, natural treatment that works.
- Dry skin? A natural moisturizing treatment that does wonders.
- How to sleep peacefully all night long.
- Angry husband? Nagging wife? Here's help for stress.
- Toxic Shock Syndrome: how to avoid it.

IT'S EASY TO ORDER

Just return this notice with your name and address and a check for **$9.95** plus $2.00 shipping and handling to our address: **FC&A, Dept. YDZ-1**, 103 Clover Green, Peachtree City, Georgia 30269. We will send you a copy of *"Encyclopedia of Natural Health Secrets and Cures"* right away.

Save! Return this notice with **$19.90+** $2.00 for two books. (No extra shipping and handling charges.)

You get a no-time-limit guarantee of satisfaction or your money back.

You must cut out and return this notice with your order. Copies wil not be accepted.!

IMPORTANT — FREE GIFT OFFER

All orders will receive a free gift. Order right away. ©FC&A

"HE DIED WITH ARTERIES LIKE A BABY"

RESEARCHERS DISCOVER EVIDENCE THAT THE HUMAN BODY HAS ITS OWN NATURAL SYSTEM THAT HELPS KEEP THE ARTERIES CLEAN

(By Frank K. Wood)

Can your arteries be cleaned out naturally? That's what many doctors are asking themselves after an autopsy of a famous nutrition expert who committed suicide.

CAN THE BODY KEEP ITS ARTERIES CLEAN?

What interests the doctors is that the "free from artery disease" theory of the nutrition expert may be proven by his death! The doctor who performed the autopsy was, in his own words "amazed to find no evidence of coronary artery disease in a man of his age (69)". He said that the nutrition expert had "arteries like a baby". What's even more amazing is that the nutrition expert was diagnosed as actually having coronary artery disease 30 years earlier when he was 39 years old.

The nutrition expert put himself on a special program to fight coronary artery disease. You'll learn about it in a new $9.95 book for the general public, *"Arteries Cleaned Out Naturally"*.

It reveals a startling new discovery by medical researchers. They say they have discovered evidence that the human body has its own natural system that helps keep the arteries clean.

Case studies like this may be atypical. There is no proof that already narrowed or clogged arteries will open up when we start to do things which might help the body's natural cleansing process.

THE AMAZING STORY OF LDL's AND HDL's

You'll learn about the new scientific discovery that the human body seems to have its own natural system which helps keep the arteries clean.

You'll learn about how LDL molecules seem to carry cholesterol into the walls of coronary arteries and lead to heart and artery disease. You'll also learn about how other molecules, HDL's, seem to play a part in the body's natural cleansing system.

The recent discoveries about HDL's are important because researchers think that most coronary artery disease is avoidable. There's a lot we can do to help keep our arteries clean.

WHAT "ARTERIES CLEANED OUT NATURALLY" REVEALS

- The amazing story of HDL's.
- The latest research evidence that the human body has its own natural system that helps keep the arteries clean.
- Four different types of heart and artery disease explained in easy-to-understand language.
- Why hardening of the arteries and high blood pressure may be higher now than years ago.
- Vitamins and minerals . . . can they help prevent artery disease?
- Exercise . . . one type that's harmful, another type that helps.
- Why some people get heart attacks even though they're health conscious.
- Heart surgery . . . when it's likely not to help . . . when relief may be obtained by other means.
- Why some fat people don't suffer from artery disease.
- Low-fat diets, are they helpful?
- Relaxation training . . . is it for you?
- Why foot problems are associated with high rates of heart attack.
- No-nonsense tips from researchers on artery cleansing.
- The smoking and heart disease connection.
- Does smoking really cause heart attacks?
- Does salt cause high blood pressure?
- How to add 10 years to your life.

IT'S EASY TO ORDER

Just return this notice with your name and address and a check for **$9.95** plus $2.00 shipping and handling to our address: **FC&A, Dept. XDZ-1,** 103 Clover Green, Peachtree City, Georgia 30269. We will send you a copy of *"Arteries Cleaned Out Naturally"* right away.

Save! Return this notice with **$19.90** + $2.00 for two books. (No extra shipping and handling charges.)

You get a no-time-limit guarantee of satisfaction or your money back.

You must cut out and return this notice with your order. Copies will not be accepted!

IMPORTANT — FREE GIFT OFFER

All orders will receive a free gift. Order right away!

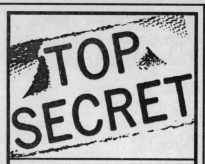

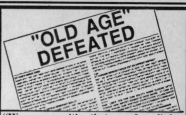

6

GLOSSARY

Each of the drugs described in detail in *Chapter 5* are noted as being in a particular **Category Of Drug.** This glossary contains definitions of each of these category terms. Also, many drug-related medical terms not found in this book are listed and defined. This chapter also includes definitions of certain common prefixes, suffixes and abbreviations often used with brand name drugs.

Anyone wanting to find out more about a particular drug should request the manufacturer's "package insert" for that drug. This can be obtained free-of-charge from a pharmacist or directly from the manufacturer. Since many of these package-inserts are written in technical medical language, this glossary should be helpful in "translating" the information leaflets.

Addiction — A state of physical dependence produced by habitually taking a drug. Physical symptoms and an overwhelming desire for the drug occur when it is withdrawn.

Adrenal Hormone — Substance produced by the body's adrenal glands; medicine may be natural or synthetic. Adrenocorticoids, like drugs made by the outer part, or cortex, of the adrenal glands, are used primarily to reduce inflammation.

Adrenocortical Hormone — See: Adrenal Hormone.

Allergy — A disorder of the body's immunity system where the body attacks foreign substances such as foods, pollens or drugs in a way which causes rashes, inflammation, or other allergic reactions in the body.

Analgesic — Pain reliever.

Anemia — A reduction in the quantity of hemoglobin or the size and number of red blood cells available for carrying oxygen throughout the body.

Anesthetic — A drug which causes loss of sensation of feeling.

Angina Pectoris — Severe chest pain, often extending down the left shoulder and arm, caused by lack of blood supply flowing through the coronary arteries to the heart.

Antacid — Substance used to neutralize excess acid in the stomach.

Anti-alcoholism Drug — To treat alcoholism by causing nausea when alcohol is consumed.

340

Anti-allergy Drug — To treat allergic symptoms such as rashes and inflammations.

Anti-arrhythmic Drugs — To regulate heartbeat or heart rhythm.

Anti-arthritic Drug — To treat the symptoms of arthritis.

Anti-asthmatic Drug — To treat the symptoms of asthma.

Antibacterial — To stop or prevent the growth of bacteria.

Antibiotic — A drug produced from a mold or other micro-organism which stops or slows the growth of other micro-organism such as bacteria.

Anticholinergic Drug — To regulate the involuntary nervous system.

Anticlotting Drug — To reduce the tendency of blood to clot.

Anticoagulant — See: Anticlotting.

Anticonvulsant — To treat or prevent violent, involuntary muscle contractions.

Anticough — To prevent excessive coughing.

Antidepressant — To treat the symptoms of mood

depression without causing overstimulation.

Antidiabetic — To treat the symptoms of diabetes mellitus.

Antidiarrhea Drug — To treat diarrhea.

Antidote — A medicine used to counteract poisonous side effects of chemicals or drugs.

Antidyskenetic — See: Antitremor.

Antiemetic — See: Antivomiting.

Antiflatulent Drug — To relieve discomfort caused by excess gas in the stomach or intestines.

Antifungus Drug — To treat fungus infections.

Antiglaucoma Drug — To treat glaucoma and excessive pressure within the eyeball.

Antihistamine — A drug with many uses including relieving allergic symptoms by inactivating, a natural substance found within the body.

Antihypertensive Drug — Blood-pressure reducer.

Anti-infective Drug — To treat infections, usually within a specific area of the body such as the urinary tract.

Anti-inflammatory Drug — To reduce

inflammation.

Anti-itching — To reduce itching.

Antilipidemic Drug — To reduce the amount of fat in the blood.

Antinausea Drug — To combat nausea.

Antiparasite — To combat parasites, such as worms, within the body.

Antiprotozoa — To combat protozoa, a micro-organism bigger than bacteria, which often causes stomach upsets and diarrhea.

Antipyretic Drug — See: Fever Reducer.

Antirheumatic Drug — To treat rheumatism or rheumatoid arthritis.

Antisenility Drug — To reduce symptoms of senility, such as loss of memory and reason.

Antispasm Drug — To reduce muscle spasms that are beyond a person's control such as stomach spasms or other involuntary spasms.

Antitoxin — A drug to neutralize the affects of toxins, which are poisons usually produced by bacteria invading the body.

Antitremor Drug — To prevent tremors or fine involuntary muscle movements as, for example, in the hands.

Antitussive Drug — To relieve coughing.

Antivirus Drug — To combat viruses.

Antivomiting Drug — To prevent vomiting.

Arrhymia — Irregular heartbeats.

Appetite Suppressant — To reduce excessive appetite.

Ataxia — Involuntary, incoordinated muscle movements.

Bacteria — Microscopic living organisms which may infect people and cause disease.

Blood Count — The number of white or red blood cells contained in a standard size sample of blood.

Blood Dyscrasia — Abnormal condition of the blood.

Blood Fat Reducer — To reduce the amount of fat circulating in the blood.

Blood Pressure Reducer — To relieve hypertension or high blood pressure.

Blood Sugar — The amount of sugar found in a standard size sample of blood.

Blood Thinner — An inaccurate term to describe drugs which reduce the tendency of blood to clot.

Blood Vessel Enlarger — A drug which enlarges blood vessels to allow greater circulation of blood.

Blood Vessel Dilator — See: Blood Vessel Enlarger.

Bradycardia — Slow heart beat.

Bronchial Tube Relaxer — A drug which relaxes or opens bronchial tubes in cases of congestion.

Bronchodilator — See: Bronchial Tube Relaxer.

Calorie — Unit of measure which determines the energy value of foods.

Carcinoma — Cancer.

Cardiac — Of or relating to the heart.

Cardiac Arrest — Heart-attack or when productive heart beating stops.

Cardiotonic — See: Heart Rhythm Regulator.

Cataract — Clouding of the lens of the eye.

Caustic — A substance which causes irritation and burning, to promote peeling of skin or remove warts.

Cholinergic — A drug affecting the regulation of the body's involuntary nervous system.

CL — Chloride form of a drug.

Coagulant Drug — To cause the blood to clot.

Coma — Unconsciousness from which a person cannot be awakened.

Congestion — An accumulation of fluid within a particular part of the body.

Constrict — To tighten or reduce diameter, as in a constricted blood vessel.

CR — Controlled release form of a drug.

Decongestant — A drug which reduces congestion.

DEMI — A smaller dosage form of a drug.

Dermatological — Referring to the skin or treatment of the skin.

Dextrose — A simple sugar.

Diabetes Mellitus — An insufficient supply of insulin produced by the body or insensitivity to insulin produced by the body which reduces the body's ability to burn or store sugar.

Dilate — To enlarge a blood vessel, or other opening, such as the pupil of the eye.

Disinfectant — A substance applied to outer surfaces to kill bacteria or other micro-organisms.

Diuretic — A drug that increases the flow of urine.

Dose — The amount of a medicine to be taken at one time or over a certain period.

Drug-dependence — Drug addiction.

Drug Interaction — One drug or other substance increasing, decreasing or changing the effects of another drug.

Drug Sensitivity — Extreme or allergic reaction to a drug.

DS — Double strength dose of a drug.

Dyspnea — Shortness of breath.

Dysuria — Difficult urination.

Edema — Accumulation of fluid in the body.

EEG — Electroencephalogram or brain wave recording.

EKG — Electrocardiogram or heart wave recording.

Electrolytes — Various types of salts found in body fluids and tissues.

Embolism — Blockage of a blood vessel by a clot or other material.

Emollient — A medicine which soothes or softens irritated mucous membranes or skin.

Endocrine Glands — Glands which produce and release hormones directly into the body without using any ducts or channels.

Enteric-Coated — Specially coated to release the drug in the intestine, must be taken whole. If crushed, they will release in the stomach and lose their unique protection.

Enzyme — A protein produced by living organisms which stimulates a chemical reaction while the enzyme remains unchanged.

Epilepsy — A disorder caused by disturbed brain impulses and characterized by convulsions, unconsciousness, or momentary lapses of consciousness.

Estrogen — A synthetic or natural hormone like that produced by the ovaries which causes female sex characteristics and plays a part in menstrual changes and other bodily processes.

Euphoria — A feeling of elation or excessive happiness, often without apparent reason.

Eustachian Tube — The tube connecting the middle ear to the pharynx (back of the throat).

Expectorant — See: Phlegm Loosener.

Fallopian Tube — Either of a pair of tubes that conduct egg cells from the ovary to the uterus.

Female Hormone — One of several hormones produced by and characteristic of female, such as estrogen or progesterone.

Fever — Body temperature above 98.6° F.

Fever Reducer — A drug which tends to lower body temperature.

Gastritis — Inflammation of the stomach.

Generic Name — The name given to the ingredient or ingredients in a drug as distinguished from brand names for drugs which may be trademarked by manufacturers.

Glucose — The principal sugar used for energy by the body.

Hallucination — Perception of something which does not exist, usually as a result of mental illness.

Heart Rhythm Regulator — A drug to regulate heartbeat or heart rhythm.

Hepatitis — Inflammation of the liver by infection or other causes.

Histamine — Substance produced naturally by the body which may be active in large amounts in allergic reactions. Various types of histamine may cause lower blood pressure, enlargement of blood vessels, and stimulation of secretions from stomach and other organs.

Hormone — A substance produced naturally by the body which leads to physical changes or increases in body activity.

Hyperacidity — Unusually large amounts of acid.

Hyperglycemia — Excess of sugar in the blood.

Hyperkalemia — Excessive potassium in the blood.

Hypersensitivity — Abnormally sensitive reaction.

Hypertension — High blood pressure.

Hyperthyroid — Excessive activity of the thyroid gland which can cause increased metabolic rate, enlargement of the thyroid gland, high blood pressure, and rapid heart rate.

Hypnotic — See: Sleeping aid.

Hypoglycemia — Low blood sugar level.

Hypokalemia — Low level of potassium in the blood.

Hypotension — Low blood pressure.

Hypothyroid — Low activity of the thyroid gland which can cause a lowered metabolic rate and loss of energy.

Immunity — Resistance to a particular disease

Jaundice — Yellowing of the skin (often caused by liver disease).

Ketonuria — A condition which may be present in diabetes which is marked by the passage of acetone or ketone bodies in the urine.

Laxative — To stimulate bowel movement or to encourage a softer or bulkier stool.

Lesion — An injury or wound.

Lethargy — Tiredness.

Malaise — Feeling of general discomfort or "unwellness".

MAO Inhibitor — A drug usually used as an antidepressant which interferes with a particular type of enzyme in the body.

Metastasis — Moving from one part of the body to another part, usually used for movement of cancer from one part of the body to another.

Migraine Headache — A severe and usually recurrent headache often accompanied by dizziness, nausea, vomiting and visual disturbances such as seeing a jagged flash of light.

Mineral Supplement — Extra inorganic nutrients for the body's needs.

Monoamine Oxidase Inhibitor — See: MAO Inhibitor.

Muscle Relaxant — Drug to ease excess muscle tension, thus reducing pain in many cases.

Narcotic — A drug to relieve pain, induce sleep or dull the senses. Long-term use of narcotics can cause addiction. Excess doses can cause unconsiousness or death.

Nervous System Regulator — A drug to regulate or "even out" the impulses in the involuntary nervous system.

Obesity — Excess fat.

Ophthalmic — Having to do with the eye.

Oral Contraceptive — A drug containing female

352

hormones, usually synthetic estrogen and progesterone, to provide birth control by inhibiting the body's natural cycle of female hormone production which interferes with ovulation or the release of eggs.

Otic — Having to do with the ear.

Over-the-Counter Drug — Medication which may be purchased without prescription.

Pain Reliever — A drug intended mainly to relieve pain.

Palpitation — Pounding heartbeat.

Pancreatic Hormone — A hormone produced by the pancreas gland.

Paralysis — Muscle weakness, partial or total.

Phlegm — Thick mucus secretions in the respiratory tract.

Phlegm Loosener — Drugs which "water down" and loosen thick phlegm.

Pill — Medicine in a small round mass.

Plasma — The fluid "watery" part of the blood.

Pneumonia — Inflammation of the lung caused by bacteria or other micro-organisms.

Polyuria — Excessive urination.

Prescription — Written directions for the preparation and taking of medicine prepared by a licensed medical practitioner, such as a physician.

Progestins — Female hormones which cause changes in the uterus to prepare it for receiving a fertilized egg — or pregnancy.

Prostatic Hypertrophy — Enlarged prostate gland.

Psychotherapeutic Drug — To treat mental or emotional disorders.

Rash — A skin eruption on the body often characterized by red spots or splotches.

Rectal Cream — A cream for application to the rectal area or anus, usually for soothing or reducing inflammation or infection.

Respiration — Breathing.

Sedative — A drug with a calming effect.

Sleeping Aid — A drug to induce or aid sleep.

Somnolence — Sleepiness.

Stimulant — A drug which stimulates the brain and

nervous system, causing greater wakefulness or attention.

Stomach Acid Secretion Inhibitor — A drug which is specific for inhibiting the secretion of stomach acid by blocking histamine (H2).

Sublingual Tablets — To be dissolved underneath the tongue. Made to be absorbed by the tiny blood vessels in the mouth. Must NOT be crushed or swallowed, but must be allowed to dissolve completely in the mouth.

Sulfa Drug — An anti-infective, diuretic or anti-diabetic drug belonging to a certain chemical group of related sulfur compounds.

Suppository — A tapered plug for insertion into the rectum.

Sympathomimetic Drug — Affects the involuntary nervous system, causing increases in blood pressure, relief of congestion and other effects.

Symptom — A change in feeling or sensation relating to a disease.

Syndrome — A group of signs and symptoms which occur together and which indicate a particular disease.

Systemic — Affecting the inner workings of the body as a whole.

Tablet — Solid form of medicine to be taken by mouth.

Tachycardia — Rapid heart beat.

Testosterone — Male sex hormone.

Timed Release — Medication which is released slowly and evenly over a long period of time. The following special types must NOT be crushed — sustained action (SA), sustained release (SR), timed release (TR), spansule, extentabs or repetabs.

Tinnitus — Actual or perceived ringing noise in the ears.

Topical — Applied locally to the area to be treated such as the skin or the eyes instead of taken internally.

Toxic — Poisonous.

Tranquilizer — To reduce tension and anxiety without excessive sedation.

Tremor — Involuntary quivering or shaking.

Tricyclic Antidepressant — To treat depression without over-stimulation. Tricyclic refers to the chemical structure of this class of drugs.

Tumor — An abnormal mass of growing tissue that is not caused by inflammation or infection. Tumors may or may not be cancerous.

Ulcer — A wound, hole, or lesion on the surface of a mucous membrane such as the lining of the stomach or other

DRUG MANUFACTURERS' ADDRESSES

The following list contains the address of each manufacturer whose brand name drugs are described in this book. It is intended to be an aid in your obtaining any additional information concerning any of these, or other, drugs.

Each manufacturer has personnel on staff who are genuinely ready to answer questions. They are also interested in receiving information from patients who are currently taking their drugs. If you experience any side effects which are not listed in their materials, have your doctor verify the condition and notify the manufacturer.

Abbott Pharmaceuticals
Abbott Park
P.O.Box 68
North Chicago, IL 60064

Adria Laboratories, Inc.
P.O. Box 16529
Columbus, OH 43216

Alcon Laboratories, Inc.
P.O. Box 1959
Fort Worth, TX 76134

Allergan Pharmaceuticals, Inc.
2525 Dupont Drive
Irvine, CA 92713

American Critical Care
Div. of Amer. Hospital Supply Corp.
McGaw Park, IL 60085

Armour Pharmaceutical Company
303 South Broadway
Tarrytown, NY 10591

Astra Pharmaceutical Products, Inc.
7 Neponset Street
Worchester, MA 01606

Ayerst Laboratories
Div. of American Home Products Corp.
685 Third Avenue
New York, NY 10017

Beecham Laboratories
Div. of Beecham, Inc.
Bristol, TN 37620

Berlex Laboratories, Inc.
Cedar Knolls, NJ 07927

Boehringer Ingelheim Ltd.
90 East Ridge
P.O.Box 368
Ridgefield, CT 06877

Boots Pharmaceuticals, Inc.
6540 Line Avenue
Shreveport, LA 71106

Breon Laboratories, Inc.
90 Park Avenue
New York, NY 10016

Bristol Laboratories
Div. of Bristol-Meyers Co.
Thompson Rd., P.O. Box 657
Syracuse, NY 13201

Burroughs Wellcome Company
3030 Cornwallis Road
Research Triangle Park, NC 27709

Burton, Parsons & Company
A Div. of Alcon Laboratories, Inc.
6201 South Freeway
Fort Worth, TX 76134

Carnrick Laboratories, Inc.
65 Horse Hills Road
Cedar Knolls, NJ 07927

CIBA Pharmaceutical Company
Div. of CIBA-GEIGY Corporation
556 Morris Avenue
Summit, NJ 07901

Coopervision Pharmaceuticals, Inc.
Medical Department
455 East Middlefield Road
Mountain View, CA 94043

Dermik Laboratories, Inc.
1777 Walton Road, Dublin Hall
Blue Bell, PA 19422

Dista Products Company
Div. of Eli Lilly and Company
Medical Department
307 East McCarty Street
Indianapolis, IN 46285

Dorsey Pharmaceuticals
Div. of Sandoz, Inc.
Medical Department
East Hanover, NJ 07936

Dow B. Hickman, Inc.
P.O.Box 35413
Houston, TX 77035

Endo Pharmaceuticals, Inc.
Subsidiary of the DuPont Company
One Rodney Square
Wilmington, DE 19898

Ex-Lax Pharmaceutical
Div. of Sandoz, Inc.
New York, NY 10158
Flint Laboratories
Div. of Travenol Laboratories, Inc.
Deerfield, IL 60015
GEIGY Pharmaceuticals
Div. of CIBA-GEIGY Corporation
Medical Services Department
Ardsley, NY 10502
Glaxo, Inc.
1900 West Commercial Blvd.
Fort Lauderdale, FL 33309
**Hoechst-Roussel
Pharmaceuticals, Inc.**
Route 202-206 North
Somerville, NJ 08876
Hoyt Laboratories
Div. of Colgate-Palmolive Co.
575 University Avenue
Norwood, MA 02062
Ives Laboratories, Inc.
685 Third Avenue
New York, NY 10017
Janssen Pharmaceutica, Inc.
501 George Street
New Brunswick, NJ 08903
Key Pharmaceuticals, Inc.
18425 NW 2nd Avenue
Miami, FL 33169
**Knoll Pharmaceutical
Company**
30 North Jefferson Road
Whippany, NJ 07981
Kremers-Urban Company
P.O. Box 2038
Milwaukee, WI 53201

Robins (A.H.) Company
Pharmaceutical Division
1407 Cummings Drive
Richmond, VA 23220

Roche Laboratories
Div. of Hoffman-La Roche, Inc.
Nutley, NJ 07110

Roerig
A Division of Pfizer Pharmaceuticals
235 E. 42nd Street
New York, NY 10017

Rorer (William H.), Inc.
500 Virginia Drive
Fort Washington, PA 19034

Ross Laboratories
Div. Abbott Laboratories
Columbus, OH 43216

Sandoz Pharmaceuticals
Div. of Sandoz, Inc.
Route 10
East Hanover, NJ 07936

Schering Corporation
Galloping Hill Road
Kenilworth, NJ 07033

Searle & Company
G.D. Searle & Company
Medical Communications Department
Box 5110
Chicago, IL 60680

Smith Kline & French Laboratories
Div. of SmithKline Beckman Corporatior
1500 Spring Garden Street
P.O. Box 7929
Philadelphia, PA 19101

Squibb (E.R.) & Sons, Inc.
General Offices
P.O. Box 4000
Princeton, NJ 08540

Stiefel Laboratories, Inc.
2801 Ponce de Leon Blvd.
Coral Gables, FL 33134

Stuart Pharmaceuticals
Div. of ICI Americas, Inc.
Wilmington, DE 19897

Syntex Laboratories, Inc.
3401 Hillview Avenue
Palo Alto, CA 94304

The Upjohn Company
7000 Portage Road
Kalamazoo, MI 49001

**USV Pharmaceutical
Corporation**
1 Scarsdale Road
Tuckahoe, NY 10707

Wallace Laboratories
P.O. Box 1
Cranbury, NJ 08512

Webcon Pharmaceuticals
Div. of Alcon, Inc.
P.O. Box 1629
Fort Worth, TX 76101

Westwood Pharmaceuticals, Inc.
468 Dewitt Street
Buffalo, NY 14213

Winthrop Laboratories
90 Park Avenue
New York, NY 10016

Wyeth Laboratories
Div. of American Home Products
P.O. Box 8299
Philadelphia, PA 19101